"Kim's book lays the groundwork for what every person should understand about inflammation and their health. We are facing diseases and conditions that stem from inflammation in epidemic proportions. Kim walks the reader through understanding the difficult topic of chronic inflammation and provides an actionable lifestyle plan for combating it. A must read for anyone who is interested in health maintenance and disease prevention."

—Whitney Ahneman, MS, RDN, CDE, CLT

"Sound nutrition advice from a nutrition expert. Filled with practical nutrition tips and tidbits, Ms. Tessmer's book is a terrific manual for anyone interested in eating their way to optimal health."

—Colleen D. Webb, MS, RDN, CLT

Praise for *Your Nutrition Solution to Inflammation*

"Kimberly's book managed to compile many of the best nutritional approaches to reducing inflammation scattered throughout literature and encapsulate them into one reference source. At the same time, the book is penned in a general, easily understood tone that can be useful to all. Main points are reiterated in 'tidbits' to facilitate learning retention. Confusing areas of nutrition are explained in detail, such as what BMI is, how it is calculated, and why it is related to inflammation. In summation, I found it to be an entertaining, comprehensive, and application-based resource for those looking for natural ways to reduce the pain and disability that results from chronic inflammation."

—Kathy J. Shattler, MS, RDN, Registered Dietitian Nutritionist, Virtual Nutritional Synergy

"*Your Nutrition Solution to Inflammation* could also be titled 'Step by Step Eating to a Healthier Life.' This book provides straightforward understandable explanations and honest nutritional information without resorting to gimmicks or fads. It is organized in a manner where each chapter builds on the previous but also stands alone. A reader could open randomly to almost any page and find a practical, doable suggestion or tip that, if implemented, would improve the reader's food choices. The tips, lists, and menu guides take all the 'shoulds' that we as dietitians teach people and transforms them into achievable 'how-to's' without being overwhelming. A must read for non-dietitians/nutritionists seeking to improve their nutritional status and a model for dietitians on how to present nutritional information in an approachable format."

—Mavis Miller RD, CSG, LD

your nutrition
SOLUTION

to

INFLAMMATION

your nutrition
SOLUTION

to

INFLAMMATION

a meal-based plan to help reduce or manage the
symptoms of autoimmune diseases, arthritis,
fibromyalgia, and more as well as decrease
risk for other serious illnesses

kimberly tessmer, RDN, LD

NEW PAGE BOOKS
A division of The Career Press, Inc.
Pompton Plains, NJ

Your Nutrition Solution to Inflammation
Edited by Roger Sheety
Original cover design by Joanna Williams
Printed in the U.S.A.

To order this title, please call toll-free 1-800-CAREER-1 (NJ and Canada: 201-848-0310) to order using VISA or MasterCard, or for further information on books from Career Press.

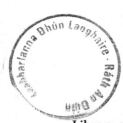

The Career Press, Inc.
220 West Parkway, Unit 12
Pompton Plains, NJ 07444
www.careerpress.com

Library of Congress Cataloging-in-Publication Data

Tessmer, Kimberly A.
    Your nutrition solution to inflammation : a meal-based plan to help reduce or manage the symptoms of autoimmune diseases, arthritis, fibromyalgia and more, as well as decrease risk for other serious illnesses / by Kimberly Tessmer, RDN, LD.
        pages cm. -- (Your nutrition solution)
    ISBN 978-1-60163-367-5 (paperback) -- ISBN 978-1-60163-385-9 (ebook)
        1. Inflammation--Diet therapy--Popular works. 2. Inflammation--Diet therapy--Recipes. 3. Inflammation--Nutritional aspects. I. Title.

RB131.T42 2015
641.5'63--dc23
                                                            2015002488

Disclaimer

At the time this book was written, all information herein was believed by the author to be correct and accurate. Information on inflammation changes frequently as more research is being completed. Always keep yourself up-to-date by reading reputable and current publications, and speaking with your healthcare provider. The author shall have no liability of any kind for damages of any nature, however caused. The author will not accept any responsibility for any omissions, misinterpretations, or misstatements that may exist within this book. The author does not endorse any product or company listed in this book. Always consult with your healthcare provider for medical advice, as well as recommendations on any type of supplement or herbal supplement you plan on taking. The author is not engaged in rendering medical services and this book should not be construed as medical advice nor should it take the place of being properly diagnosed and monitored by your regular healthcare provider.

Dedication

I dedicate this book to all of the people that deal daily with chronic inflammation and its consequences. My hope is that this book will be able to help you in some way to relieve the pain and frustration that goes along with dealing with daily chronic inflammation. Allow this book to empower you to make the necessary changes needed to start feeling better and managing your health for a lifetime. I am always grateful to be able to dedicate my books to my Dad and to my late Mom, who I miss dearly. I am so thankful for the gift they passed on to me for helping others. That is what gives me my passion to be a dietitian and help others deal with their struggles.

Acknowledgments

A loving thank-you to my wonderful husband, Greg, who works so hard, which allows me to do what I love, and to my daughter, Tori, who is always patient and gives Mommy the time to do her writing. I would like to thank all of my fellow RDs who gave me their expert input and advice on this subject. A special thank you to Whitney Ahneman, MS, RDN, CLT and all of the other dietitians who took time out of their busy schedule to review my book and provide endorsements.

contents

introduction

The word "inflammation" tends to conjure up all types of images in your head including redness, pain, swelling, and heat. These can all be the case with acute inflammation. When you fall off your bike and scrape your knee or cut yourself with a knife, the site of the injury normally shows symptoms of acute inflammation, including all of the descriptive words we just used. This is your body's natural immune and protective response to tissue damage. That redness, pain, swelling, and feeling of being inflamed are all good signs that your body's immune system is doing what it should and sending white blood cells to the affected area to repair the damaged tissue.

Although we will discuss both types of inflammation, the type that the majority of this book will encompass is called *chronic* or *systemic inflammation,* which can seriously affect one's health and possibly be the root cause for many health issues. In fact, chronic inflammation may be responsible for more health issues in this country than we even realize. For some people, the inflammation response is triggered inappropriately and/or never shuts off once it is triggered. This leads to chronic inflammation, which continually drains energy from the body, in turn weakening the immune system and making it vulnerable to the triggering of other health conditions.

Research has found that the effects of this invisible but chronic inflammation may play a role in the aging process and in age-related diseases such as heart disease, arthritis, asthma, diabetes, certain types of cancer, Parkinson's, Alzheimer's, and autoimmune disease, just to name a few. It is believed that genetics may play a role in your risk for chronic inflammation. However, the good news is that it is also believed that lifestyle and diet can make a difference and we have total control over both of these. This book will help you to find out how to change your diet and lifestyle to help fight against chronic inflammation now and in the future. It is time to take charge of your own health and this book *is* your nutrition solution to inflammation!

chapter 1

your questions about inflammation, answered

The word "inflammation" is one of the newest medical buzz words. And with good reason! Inflammation has become a huge area of interest to medical researchers as they are beginning to discover that it may play a critical role in the occurrence of many chronic health conditions and diseases. Not all inflammation is bad, and we will find out more about what it actually is and the difference between acute and chronic inflammation in this chapter.

What Is the Difference Between Acute and Chronic Inflammation?

Although the word "inflammation" may not always conjure up the best thoughts, not all inflammation is entirely bad. *Acute inflammation* is part of the body's immune response and the body's attempt to protect itself from infection and further harm. For example, if you have an injury such as a cut or scrape on your skin or you take a blow to your knee, or even if you have a bacterial infection in your lungs such as bronchitis, the

signs and symptoms of inflammation display a biological response by the body to remove harmful stimuli and begin the
healing process. During the inflammation process, the body
produces white blood cells and other substances to protect itself from foreign organisms. Cuts, wounds, infections, and
damage to tissue would not heal without acute inflammation.
Acute inflammation comes on quick, is short-lasting, and is a
very normal and necessary process to help protect our body. In
this case, it's a good thing.

Your Nutrition Solution Tidbit

Inflammation does not always mean an infection is
present. An infection is normally caused by bacteria, a virus, or fungus, whereas acute inflammation
is the body's response to that specific infection.

On the flip side of the inflammation coin is *chronic inflammation*, which is a whole other story. This type of inflammation
is long-lasting and ongoing, from several months to years, and
plays a more puzzling role in the body. Chronic inflammation
can occur from acute inflammation that has a persistent stimulus and/or when your body loses the ability to turn off the acute
inflammatory response and the inflammation then begins to
damage healthy tissue and cells without foreign invaders present. Chronic inflammation can be caused from an autoimmune
response as well, which can damage many parts of the body
from your digestive system to your heart to your joints. The
body basically responds as if healthy tissue is infected or ab-
normal, even though it is not. The problem occurs when chronic inflammation eventually affects the healthy tissue, causing
or becoming the root problem in many health conditions and
diseases.

Your Nutrition Solution Tidbit

Chronic inflammation is also sometimes referred to as *systemic inflammation,* which happens when inflammation moves beyond the affected tissues and into the lining of the blood vessels and organs. This can seriously affect your health and cause a host of health issues.

What Health Conditions and Diseases Are Associated With Inflammation?

There are a wide variety of health issues that are associated with both acute and chronic inflammation. In addition, there are many autoimmune disorders that can cause the body's immune system to mistakenly initiate an inflammatory response even though there is nothing to fight off.

Examples of health conditions that are associated with *acute inflammation* include:

- Acute bronchitis.
- Infected ingrown toe nail.
- A cut or bump.
- Sore throat.
- Acute sinusitis.
- Acute tonsillitis.
- Acute appendicitis.
- Stuffy nose.
- Sprained ankle.
- Burn to the skin.

The development of a specific health condition depends on the particular site where the inflammatory response occurs. For example, if the response or disruption occurs in the intestinal cells, this can lead to inflammatory bowel disease (IBD), including Crohn's Disease or ulcerative colitis. Although different health conditions and diseases will have different underlying factors that might trigger it, the mechanism that links chronic inflammation and disease is evidenced by the same progression.

Examples of health conditions that are associated with chronic inflammation that are inflammatory by nature or an autoimmune disorder include:

- Asthma.
- Rheumatoid arthritis.
- Inflammatory bowel disease, such as ulcerative colitis and Crohn's disease.
- Irritable bowel syndrome (IBS).
- Lupus.
- Fibromyalgia (often a set of symptoms associated with another autoimmune disorder).
- Chronic sinusitis.
- Tendonitis.
- Diverticulitis (can also be associated with acute inflammation).
- Gingivitis.
- Gluten sensitive conditions/celiac disease.
- Psoriasis.
- Atherosclerosis/heart disease.
- Type 2 diabetes/insulin resistance.
- Hashimoto's thyroiditis.

Additionally, there are other health issues that researches are now finding may have chronic inflammation as their root cause, including atherosclerosis/heart disease, hypertension, metabolic syndrome, obesity, certain types of cancer, allergies, gallbladder disease, non-alcoholic fatty liver disease, and maybe even Alzheimer's disease. Heart disease is the number-one killer for Americans, but did you know that one of the biggest causes of heart disease is inflammation? Inflammation can also trigger an increase in the "bad" cholesterol or low density lipoproteins (LDL), which are a major risk factor for heart disease. You can change your diet and lifestyle to lower cholesterol, or even take medications, but if you don't get to the root cause of chronic inflammation, you won't get to the bottom of the problem in order to solve it. It is quite the domino effect. That is where our diet comes in. The greatest source of inflammation for most Americans is their everyday diet, whether they have a poor diet or hidden food sensitivities and intolerances. And that is something we all have control over.

Is Fibromyalgia an Inflammation-Related Disorder?

Fibromyalgia syndrome is a chronic disorder that in general causes widespread muscle and joint pain, painful tender points, crippling fatigue, and a number of other harsh symptoms including depression. It is one of the most common musculoskeletal conditions after osteoarthritis, especially for women, and most experts tend to group it with arthritis-related disorders even though it is not truly a form of arthritis. However, fibromyalgia is considered a rheumatic condition, which is a medical disorder that impairs the joints and/or soft tissue and causes chronic pain. It does not cause inflammation and damage to joints as arthritis does.

The cause of this disorder is still unclear. It may deal with genes and run in families, and it most often materializes due to a triggering factor, many times rheumatic in nature, such as lupus, osteoarthritis, and/or rheumatoid arthritis. Even though fibromyalgia does cause inflammation, much of the way it is treated and dealt with is the same as methods for helping to reduce inflammation including medications, exercise, sleep habits, relaxation, and possibly diet. The benefits of adding or avoiding specific foods can be different for every individual, so keeping a food diary can be extremely helpful in identifying personal triggers for pain and also for which foods might make you feel better. Following the tips in this book can possibly help and surely can't hurt.

What Causes Inflammation?

When acute inflammation occurs, chemicals from our body's white blood cells are released into the bloodstream and/or affected tissues to protect that area from foreign substances. The release of chemicals in turn increases the blood flow to the area, which usually results in the redness, swelling, and warmth that you feel when you have inflammation. The whole process, though protective, can sometimes cause pain by stimulating nerves.

Chronic inflammation, as we mentioned before, can be related to the failure of the body to eliminate whatever was causing the acute inflammation or the presence of a persistent stimulus causing acute inflammation to evolve into chronic inflammation. This stimulus can be a host of free radicals that come from highly processed foods we eat every day, it could be an allergy or intolerance to gluten or other food substances which in turn inflames the lining of the gut, or a low-grade lingering infection that we are not even aware of. Chronic inflammation can also be caused by an autoimmune response—basically your immune system attacking your healthy cells and tissue, mistaking them for something that is harmful even though they are not. The pain in chronic inflammation, such as in a joint, can be caused by an increased number of cells and inflammatory substances within the area that cause irritation and swelling. In the example of the joint, the swelling of the joint lining eventually wears down the cartilage, which is the cushioning at the end of the bones, causing pain.

Other possible inflammation triggers can include obesity, anxiety, food allergies, hormonal changes, poor diet, lack of sleep, and stress—just to name a few.

How Do Food Allergies/Intolerances/ Sensitivities Affect Inflammation?

Food allergies, intolerances, and sensitivities can often be an overlooked cause of chronic inflammation. We mentioned previously that a good majority of inflammatory issues for Americans are a direct result of their everyday diet. This can be from a poor diet, from hidden food intolerances; allergies; sensitivities or from a combination of these. Many inflammatory conditions such as celiac disease, inflammatory bowel disease (ulcerative colitis and Crohn's disease), IBS, and arthritis, for example, are linked to dietary factors or foods that either seem to cause or exacerbate symptoms of inflammation. Well over 50 percent of our immune cells are found in our digestive tract. If the immune system becomes triggered and/or confused by hidden food allergens and intolerances, it can in turn trigger chronic inflammation and weaken the immune system leaving you susceptible to numerous health conditions including autoimmune diseases.

The list of the more common food offenders can be quite long, but foods at the top of the list can include dairy products, wheat, gluten, yeast, eggs, soy, corn, food additives, and more. The problem is that people often don't even realize that a food allergy or intolerance is at the root of their inflammatory-related health issue. Further, many don't realize that their health issue is related to chronic inflammation. So how do you go about finding out if you have possible food allergies or intolerances that are causing you problems?

If you suspect you may have food sensitivities, intolerances, or allergies, you should see your doctor who can refer you to a board-certified allergist for testing, evaluation, and diagnosis. It is best not to try to diagnose a food allergy or intolerance on your own without professional guidance. Self-diagnosis can lead to unnecessary dietary restrictions, inadequate nutrition (especially in children), and a lot of unneeded frustration. It can make your health issues last longer and maybe become worse. An allergist will usually begin with a thorough medical history to determine if it is actually a food allergy or intolerance that may be causing your symptoms. Secondly, they will conduct a number of tests to help identify the possible food culprit. These might include a skin prick test, blood test, oral food challenge, and trial elimination diet. Once a discovery is made, the allergist should refer you to a registered dietitian nutritionist for further instruction on how to handle your diet in order to eliminate the food or foods that are causing you problems.

Another way to find out whether you are suffering with food sensitivities is called a Mediator Release Test (MRT). An MRT is a blood test that measures your immune reaction or sensitivity to a whole host of foods, additives, chemicals, and more. With the results of the MRT, your healthcare practitioner is able to identify a list of foods that you may be sensitive to and may be causing chronic inflammation that you are not even aware of. An MRT has been shown to have the highest level of accuracy of any food sensitivity blood test. This type of testing can often help to identify culprits that a person cannot figure out any other way. The "hub" of the immune system is the gut, and when someone consumes a food that they have a reaction or sensitivity to, the immune system sends out chemical mediators such as histamine, cytokines, and prostaglandins, which can produce chronic inflammation and damaging effects on body tissues and cause the development of symptoms and major health problems. Depending on the types of mediators released, different areas of the body are affected. For example, for some people consuming an affected food will cause migraines, for others arthritis or maybe acid reflux. Identifying the harmful substance is the first step toward improving the inflammation that results from a food sensitivity and in turn improves and impacts your long-term health. The next step involves following an individualized LEAP eating plan.

Many of you have probably never heard of LEAP (lifestyle, eating, and performance), but this could be your answer to finding out once and for all what foods and beverages are truly triggering chronic inflammation in your body. LEAP is an effective protocol that combines the MRT with the professional skills of a Certified LEAP Therapist (CLT). The CLT is able to produce a patient-specific anti-inflammatory diet dependent on the results of your MRT test to reduce inflammation and therefore reduce symptoms of health issues related to chronic inflammation. The two go hand-in-hand and have had substantial results for many individuals. A Certified LEAP Therapist, usually a dietitian, has received advanced clinical training in adverse food reactions, including food allergies, food sensitivities, and food intolerance. They know exactly how to assist clients with their LEAP Diet Protocols that are based directly on the results of their MRT blood test.

Most people who have MRT testing done along with counseling from a CLT have experienced significant improvement within the first 10 days or sooner with symptoms continuing to improve throughout the next four to six weeks. Many people experience complete symptom resolution once their triggers are identified and eliminated, depending on how closely they follow their LEAP protocol, whether they have underlying conditions involved, and to which degree food sensitivity plays a role in their condition.

If you are interested in LEAP and MRT testing, visit *http://nowleap.com* or call 1-888-Now-LEAP (toll free). You can Google "Certified LEAP Therapist" in your state, city, or zip code. In addition, there is a list of RD and RDNs in the resource section of this book to help get you started. Many will counsel via phone, so you don't need to reside in the same area. This process is definitely more than just being tested! Most people who are tested without counseling from a CLT do not do nearly as well. Talk to your doctor about being tested for food sensitivities and if you decide it is right for you, do it the correct way and partner it with a Certified LEAP Therapist. What you do with the test results is the most important step in success with this process.

Your Nutrition Solution Tidbit

A true food allergy is much less common and leads to an immune system reaction that can affect numerous organs in the body and in some cases cause severe symptoms. A food intolerance is generally less serious and is often limited to less severe symptoms such as digestive issues, headaches, and heartburn. Food intolerances occur when an individual is not able to properly digest a specific food item or when a food item causes irritation in the digestive system. A food sensitivity seems to be the most difficult to diagnose and generally means that an individual has a negative reaction to certain food items that do not always occur in the same way. Someone with a food sensitivity may be able to consume a specific food without any apparent symptoms, but will intermittently show symptoms such as acid reflux, headaches, abdominal cramps, nausea, and other digestive issues without knowing why.

What Are the Symptoms of Inflammation?

The symptoms of acute inflammation are much different than those of chronic inflammation. Symptoms of acute inflammation are usually pretty obvious and can include things such as pain, redness, swelling, heat, and joint stiffness. Acute inflammation can also include less obvious symptoms such as fever, chills, fatigue, headache, and muscle stiffness. Symptoms of chronic inflammation are not always so apparent. Most of the time, chronic inflammation is silent and you don't know there is a problem until multiple health conditions begin to emerge. Even at that point, most people do not know that inflammation is the underlying cause of their condition(s) unless it is an obvious inflammatory-related disease such as arthritis.

Can Inflammation Be Diagnosed?

The diagnosis of inflammation is only made after careful evaluation of many factors including a complete medical history, diet history, physical exam with attention to joint pain and stiffness, evaluation of other physical symptoms, as well as results of X rays and blood tests. The blood test most widely used to measure levels of inflammation in the bloodstream is called C-reactive protein (CRP). CRP is a protein made by the body from the pro-inflammatory cytokine interleukin-6 (IL-6), which is produced mainly by the liver. The level of this protein tends to increase with increased levels of inflammation. A CRP test is sometimes used to evaluate a person's risk for developing coronary artery disease (CAD) in which the arteries of the heart are narrowed. CAD can eventually lead to having a heart attack. The CRP blood test is also used to measure changes in the body's overall inflammation levels to help healthcare practitioners track progress and success of treatment. This usually occurs when a person has a health condition known to be related to inflammation such as inflammatory bowel disease, arthritis, lupus, etc. or when a person has recently had a heart attack or surgery, to check for infection. Though CRP is widely used, not all healthcare professionals agree whether it is a true sign of increased risk of disease due to inflammation.

Although CRP levels are a better indicator, erythrocyte sedimentation rate (ESR) is another test that reflects the degree of inflammation in the body. It is not able to point to a specific disease, but in healthy people the ESR is low and rises with inflammation. Both of these tests can be used to monitor both disease activity and how well someone is responding to treatment.

Your Nutrition Solution Tidbit

Should you be tested? The answer to that will be at the discretion of your doctor. However, if you find that you have multiple health issues such as type 2 diabetes, gum disease, obesity, excessive hunger, fatigue, brittle nails, headaches, are a smoker, are sedentary, are constipated, have difficulty concentrating, or experience other unexplained symptoms, you may want to speak with your doctor about inflammation, testing, and your possible risks.

What Parts of the Body Can Inflammation Affect?

Chronic inflammation is not picky. It can cause problems in all sorts of areas of the body. It can affect internal organs such as the heart, kidneys, and lungs as well as joints, skin, and gums, for instance. It can create a snowball-type effect where the inflammation flares up and evolves into a health condition with that condition evolving into another. For example, we know that obesity and type 2 diabetes often go hand in hand. Why is that? Mainly because obesity, with its extra-large fat cells, churns out more inflammatory compounds. Inflammation in turn promotes insulin resistance, which in turn promotes type 2 diabetes. It is vital to think of chronic inflammation being the root cause for certain health issues and to change factors such as weight, diet, and lifestyle that we have control over to stop the cycle and restore health before things get out of hand.

Who Is at Risk for Inflammation?

Just about anyone can be at risk for chronic inflammation, however there are some people that may be more prone to it than others. For example, people that experience repeated or prolonged infections, that smoke, that are sedentary or unfit, that are sleep deprived, have food allergies or sensitivities, or those who have gum disease can be more prone to chronic inflammation. In addition, people who are obese also have a much higher risk of experiencing chronic inflammation. People who carry excess body fat have more white blood cells (inflammatory markers) as well as more inflammatory proteins called cytokines that are churned out or that leak from fat cells. When a person gains weight, their fat cells become larger as they fill with more fat. These fat cells are stretched to their limit and can leak. Immune cells, called "macrophages," come in to save the day and clean up. However, these macrophages in turn release more inflammatory chemicals that can result in being the catalyst behind many of the negative effects being overweight or obese can have on health.

Being obese or overweight will increase your risk for chronic inflammation; but even more significant is body fat distribution or where your body stores most of your fat. If you are more of an apple shape and store more of your fat in your mid-section and abdominal area, you could be at even higher risk for the negative effects of chronic inflammation. Obesity, especially around the abdomen, is associated with chronic low-grade inflammation. Inflammation caused by excess fat in this area can lead to insulin resistance as well as other elements of metabolic syndrome, such as high blood cholesterol levels and high triglycerides. Although just about anyone is at risk for chronic inflammation, it has been clearly established that those who exhibit poor eating and lifestyle habits tend to have a higher risk for inflammation as well as higher levels of inflammation. On the flip side, those that lose weight have a decreased risk and lower levels of inflammation.

Your Nutrition Solution Tidbit

We mentioned an elevation of white blood cells as well as cytokines (a type of protein) as inflammatory markers or determinants for inflammation. Pro-inflammatory cytokines include IL-6, TNF-alpha (a), and IL-1beta (b).

How Is Inflammation Treated?

Unfortunately, when a person exhibits known inflammation, the first form of treatment tends to be medication. Over-the-counter (OTC) medications such as non-steroidal anti-inflammatory drugs (NSAIDs) like aspirin, ibuprofen, and naproxen are commonly used to help relieve pain and control inflammation. In addition to OTC medications, there are also prescription strength NSAIDs available. Most of these medications work to inhibit specific enzymes that catalyzes the formation of pro-inflammatory chemicals. However, when taken regularly for long periods of time, the risks for issues such as gastrointestinal (GI) bleeding, decreased blood clotting, and liver issues can be a major concern, and so should be discussed with your doctor first.

There are also many prescription anti-inflammatory medications that are used to treat the pain and symptoms of chronic inflammation. Again, just as with any medication taken on a regular basis, the risks need to be weighed carefully. Some prescription medications that are used for controlling inflammation may have low gastrointestinal risks but have been found to possibly increase the risk of cardiovascular events. Corticosteroids, specifically prednisone, are still another form of treatment in the fight against chronic inflammation. They are a powerful anti-inflammatory drug and are often used to treat different forms of arthritis, lupus, asthma, and other inflammatory conditions. Although these corticosteroids can be an effective tool, like many other medications, they too can have many side effects of concern when taken long term. Side effects depend greatly on the dose of medication you are taking, but in some cases they can suppress or weaken the immune system, cause bone loss, and trigger cataracts as well as cause weight gain, mood swings, elevate blood pressure, and initiate glaucoma.

To minimize side effects, your doctor may try a low-dose, short-term steroid or try other medications in combination with the steroid to help keep steroid use as low as possible. If you need to be on steroids long-term, you should discuss with your doctor ways to battle side effects such as lowering calorie intake, taking supplements for bone health, and having regular eye exams. The goal should be to find long-lasting solutions that won't be of concern, including diet and lifestyle. Once on steroids, it is important to wean off of them slowly to prevent short-term side effects.

Much needs to be considered when developing a treatment plan for someone with chronic inflammation. The good news is there are other avenues to take, either in addition to or in place of OTC and/or prescription medications. Diet, lifestyle, stress relief, body weight, certain foods, certain vitamins and minerals, and herbal and supplements may all have a very positive impact on inflammation. We will be discussing all of these throughout this book.

Are There Long-Term Complications Due to Inflammation?

Unfortunately, there are countless complications that can result from chronic inflammation. The dangerous part of chronic inflammation is that many of us don't even know it is simmering inside our body until it ignites and surfaces into a chronic medical condition. Chronic inflammation can possibly be at the root of many medical conditions with research just scratching the surface. All we can do is try to control the factors we do have control of in order to keep inflammation from ever starting in our body and to lower any inflammation that has already progressed to ensure better health.

chapter 2

the nutrition connection and beyond

Now that you have a better understanding of exactly what inflammation is, especially chronic inflammation, we can begin to take a deeper look at the nutrition connection and how it can act as a large part of the solution to managing and eliminating inflammation. This chapter will discuss significant nutrients including fats, carbohydrates, and specific vitamins and minerals, and the role they can play in helping to reduce inflammation. This chapter will also discuss even more natural ways of abolishing inflammation including dietary and herbal supplements as well as probiotics. It will help you to understand that your daily dietary intake can be the very connection that is causing your inflammation and, therefore, may be the solution to solving it.

Focusing on Fats

There are countless foods in the typical American diet that can help to eliminate or reduce chronic inflammation and those that do their part to aggravate inflammation. The type of

fat we eat is just one example. We will discuss the fats you want
to ditch and the ones you want to include.

Ditching the Unhealthy Fats

Most of us can agree that certain types of fats are not good
for our waistline or our hearts, but did you know that some
can even contribute to chronic inflammation? Some of the unhealthy fats that can have pro-inflammatory effects include
saturated fats, trans fat, and omega-6 fatty acids. In moderate
amounts, saturated fats don't tend to be much of a problem for
inflammation, but when consumed in excess, this unhealthy
fat can become an inflammatory nightmare. On the other
hand, trans fat in any amount is a problem for both health and
inflammation.

Saturated Fats

Saturated fats are most definitely one of the bad guys when
it comes to our health, especially our heart health. They are
one of the main causes of high blood cholesterol levels, even
more so than dietary cholesterol itself. Because many of these
foods are also high in cholesterol, they can become a double
whammy! Saturated fat triggers the liver to make more LDL or
"bad" cholesterol. Panel studies have shown an increased risk
for heart disease and stroke, as well as some types of cancer
when a diet is much higher in saturated fats. Saturated fats are
found primarily in animal-based foods, such as meat, the skin
on poultry, butter, and high-fat products. In addition, many
baked goods, as well as fried foods, carry high levels of saturated fat. Even though most vegetable oils are a bigger source
of unsaturated fat, there are a few plant oils that are more saturated, such as coconut, palm, and palm kernel oils. Note, however, that unrefined coconut and palm oils may also contain

strong anti-inflammatory compounds as well. The strongest link to inflammation through saturated fats is with the total amount that you consume each day. Saturated fat mostly becomes inflammatory and a problem when eaten in more than moderate amounts and on a regular basis, which unfortunately is common in the typical American diet. Many experts agree that chronic inflammation plays a bigger role in the health problems that saturated fats are blamed for. Because saturated fat is not good for our overall health, as well as heart health and inflammation, it is best to limit these as a fat source in the diet.

Your Nutrition Solution Tidbit

Grain-fed meat can be high in other pro-inflammatory compounds and low in anti-inflammatory ones. Your best bet is to choose meat that is labeled as grass-fed or pastured meat.

Trans Fatty Acids

Trans fat is by far the worse type of fat. Trans fat is created when a liquid vegetable oil is made more solid by the addition of hydrogen through a process called *hydrogenation*. These more solid fats gained popularity with manufacturers because they increase the shelf-life and flavor of many baked and processed foods. Trans fat has received more attention lately because researchers are finding out just how dangerous they can be to our health. Trans fat raises LDL (bad) cholesterol and lower HDL (good) cholesterol. In fact, they may raise LDL cholesterol even more than saturated fats and dietary cholesterol do. Consuming these fats will increase your risk for heart disease and stroke and are also associated with a higher risk for developing type 2 diabetes.

As far as inflammation goes, trans fat is highly inflammatory. It has been shown to increase C-reactive protein (CRP), which is produced by the liver and rises when there is inflammation in the body. These fats have also been shown to increase pro-inflammatory cytokines, the key regulators in inflammatory response. In January 2006, the FDA required that all manufactures begin adding "trans fat" amounts to their Nutrition Facts Panel on food labels to make it easier for consumers to know just how much trans fat they are eating. With this change, many manufacturers began taking trans fat out of their products. However, if the trans fat has been removed, it has most likely been replaced with another type of fat such as saturated fat, so check the Nutrition Facts Panel.

Most experts agree that the less trans fat you eat, the better for overall health, including inflammation. The American Heart Association recommends limiting the amount of trans fat you consume to less than 1 percent of your total daily calories. If you need 2,000 calories per day, that means getting no more than 20 of those calories from trans fats, which is less than 2 grams a day. You can decrease the amount of trans fat you eat by including more fruits, vegetables, whole grains, and fat-free or low-fat dairy products and including leaner cuts of meat, poultry without the skin, fish and seafood, legumes, nuts, and seeds. Foods highest in trans fats include fried foods, commercially baked goods, certain stick margarines, fast foods such as french fries, and some snack foods such as crackers and chips.

Your Nutrition Solution Tidbit

Even products that state "trans-fat free" can have up to 0.5 grams of trans fat per serving by labeling law definitions. This can add up quickly, especially if you are eating more than one serving. Even if the label states "trans-fat free," take a look at the ingredient list for "hydrogenated oil" or "partially hydrogenated oil" to see if the product really contains any trans fats.

Dietary Cholesterol

Even though dietary cholesterol is not an actual fat, it is worth discussing because of its possible role in inflammation and cardiovascular disease. Though it has not been thoroughly proven as of yet that there is a direct correlation between inflammation and heart disease, including heart attack and stroke, it seems to be a common denominator in people with cardiovascular disease. So if cholesterol is not a fat, what is it? Cholesterol is a waxy substance that is found in the fats (or lipids) in your blood. This compound is found only in animal foods such as meat, eggs, cheese, milk, and poultry. Although we do get cholesterol from these foods, our liver produces all we need, so it is not necessary to consume dietary cholesterol sources. Cholesterol does play an important role in the body, but it is when we have excess circulating in the blood that problems can occur. Our body needs cholesterol for some very major functions including making hormones, bile acids, and vitamin D.

In addition, cholesterol is part of every body cell. With all that we get from foods and from what our body produces, the unused excess gets stored as plaque in the arteries, increasing the risk for heart disease and stroke. When we consume high levels of dietary cholesterol, as well as saturated fat and trans fat, excess low-density lipoproteins (LDL), or the "bad" cholesterol, begins to build up in the inner walls of the arteries. Furthermore, it triggers an inflammatory response that speeds up the whole process of accumulation of LDL cholesterol on the artery walls. Like a vicious cycle, this in turn produces more inflammation. Eventually the LDL on the artery walls hardens into plaque that can rupture and lead to heart attack, stroke, and even blood clots. It goes without saying that not only should you be keeping an eye on your saturated and trans fat intake, but on your cholesterol as well.

Your Nutrition Solution Tidbit

The American Heart Association recommends keeping your intake of dietary cholesterol to less than 300 mg per day for people without coronary heart disease (CHD), and/or healthy adults, and to less than 200 mg per day for people with CHD.

Omega-6 Fatty Acids

Omega-6 fatty acids are polyunsaturated fats that are considered essential fats because our body cannot produce them and we must get them from the foods we eat. These fats are necessary in our diet for vital functions including maintaining the roles of cells, the brain, and nerves. When unsaturated fats are consumed in moderation and used to replace saturated fats or trans fats in the diet, they can help reduce total cholesterol, lower LDL (bad) blood cholesterol levels, and lower blood triglyceride levels thus lowering the risk for heart disease and stroke. Omega-6 fats are not always considered "unhealthy" and we do need them. However, they can become pro-inflammatory when consumption greatly exceeds that of omega-3 fats and a major imbalance occurs.

Although there are different types of omega-6 fats, the most common sources are in the form of linoleic acid contained in certain types of plant oils including sunflower, safflower, soybean, corn, and cottonseed. All of these contain the most omega-6 fatty acids and, except for soybean oil, are basically devoid of omega-3 fatty acids, which can cause an imbalance. The problem is that these oils are the most frequently used oils in processed foods, which Americans have increased their consumption of. They are included in mayonnaise, salad dressings, and any food made with the oils mentioned previously. In turn, this has resulted in a ratio that is much heavier on the omega-6 side than the omega-3 side. This skew in the ratio of these two fats has been associated with an increased risk for chronic inflammatory diseases that include rheumatoid arthritis, IBD, cardiovascular disease, and atherosclerosis. The linoleic acid in omega-6 fatty acids is converted in our livers to another fatty acid called "arachadonic acid." Arachadonic fatty acids are converted into pro-inflammatory eicosanoids. It is not enough to simply add more omega-3 fats to your diet because the typical person tends to consume so many omega-6 fats through processed food. The best solution is to not only increase omega-3 fats in your diet, but to also decrease omega-6 fats by reducing the amount of processed foods you consume. This should help to provide a healthier ratio between the two.

Including the Healthy Fats

The good news is that not all fats are bad! There are some fats in our diets that we need and that can have a positive impact on both our health and on chronic inflammation. Two of these fats include omega-3 fatty acids and monounsaturated fats.

Omega-3 Fatty Acids

Omega-3 fatty acids are also a group of polyunsaturated fatty acids and are an essential fat. They stand on their own as a healthy fat because of the countless health benefits they provide. These fats play a crucial role in brain function as well as normal growth and development of the body. Research shows that omega-3 fatty acids help to reduce inflammation and may help reduce the risk for heart disease, certain cancers, and arthritis, just to name a few. These heart healthy fats help lower total cholesterol, increase HDL (good) cholesterol, lower triglycerides, lower blood pressure, help alleviate some of the symptoms of depression as well as other psychological disorders, improve skin disorders, and the list goes on as more research is completed. Both the American Diabetes Association and the American Heart Association advocate eating fatty fish at least two times per week as a safe and effective way to obtain the heart healthy benefits of omega-3 fats.

Omega-3 fatty acids are found mostly in fatty fish such as salmon, herring, tuna, mackerel, and sardine, in the form of EPA (eicosapentaeonic) and DHA (docoshexaeonic), which are shown to have the most powerful effect as an anti-inflammatory compound. When our diet contains plenty of omega-3 fats, particularly those from fatty fish, our body actively reduces the amount of omega-6 fatty acid it creates, which reduces the amount of pro-inflammatory eicosanoids formed. Eicosanoids are compounds that play a major role in regulating our inflammatory response, and when we have an excess amount of them in our body, they tend to produce more of a pro-inflammatory state versus that of an anti-inflammatory state. So the more omega-3 fats we consume, the less potent the eicosanoids and the better balanced our immune response is. Omega-3 fatty acids also reduce the production of other pro-inflammatory markers including cytokines, TNF-alpha, and IL-6. In addition, these powerful fats in the form of EPA and DHA can be converted into compounds that inhibit pro-inflammatory signaling.

Omega-3 fatty acids can also be found in a variety of plant foods such as walnuts, soybeans, chia seeds, flaxseeds, pumpkin seeds, olive oil, and numerous nut oils in the form of ALA (alpha linolenic acid). However, the anti-inflammatory effects of ALA are not quite as strong as those of EPA and DHA, mentioned previously. Our body does covert ALA into EPA and DHA, but the conversion is not as effective, so you need quite a bit of ALA to get enough EPA and DHA to be beneficial.

The key is to not only incorporate more of these healthy omega-3 fats into your regular diet, but to eat them in place of the unhealthier fats. Don't go overboard though! Too much omega-3, especially in the form of supplements, can have health implications for some people. Speak with your doctor first before starting an omega-3 fish oil supplement.

Your Nutrition Solution Tidbit

New foods on the market today are fortified with omega-3 fatty acids (usually in the form of ALA) such as eggs, yogurt, peanut butter, bread, and pasta. These fortified foods usually contain very little of this healthy fatty acid, and you would need to eat a lot of the food to get close to what is recommended. Additional omega-3 fatty acids found in these foods aren't harmful, but you shouldn't substitute these "functional foods" for ones that naturally contain omega-3 fatty acids.

Monounsaturated Fatty Acids

Monounsaturated fats are as essential to the proper functioning of our body as that of polyunsaturated fats. When monounsaturated fats are used to replace saturated or trans fats, they can help to lower total cholesterol and LDL (bad) blood cholesterol, reducing the risk for heart disease and stroke. Research has shown that these fats can help to reduce inflammation and possibly protect against some types of anti-inflammatory health conditions. In addition, they can help to increase insulin sensitivity, helping the body to better utilize glucose or blood sugar. Foods highest in monounsaturated fatty acids include olive oil and olives; canola and peanut oil; sunflower and sesame oil; avocados; nuts, including hazelnuts, macadamia nuts, almonds, Brazil nuts, cashews, and pecans; and seeds, including sesame seeds and pumpkin seeds.

Tips to Controlling Your Fat Intake

The type of fat you consume can have a definite impact on triggering inflammation in your body. The key is to reduce the unhealthy fats and increase the healthy ones. Here are a few tips to help you better balance your fat intake:

- Select lean cuts of meat including skinless poultry, lean pork, and lean red meats, and watch portion size. Choose fish, seafood, and plant-based proteins such as soy foods and legumes more often than meats, especially red meats.
- When preparing foods, stick with baking, broiling, grilling, roasting, or boiling instead of frying.
- Choose low-fat or fat-free dairy products.
- Use low-fat, vegetable-based cooking spray when preparing.

- Use heart healthy liquid vegetable oils that contain more omega-3 fatty acids than omega-6 fatty acids such as extra virgin olive oil or canola oil for cooking, dressings or as a substitute for butter and margarine.

- Create your own salad dressings instead of using commercial dressings that can often be overly processed and full of saturated fats and sugar. Mix extra virgin olive oil, vinegar, and your favorite herbs and spices for a quick and healthy dressing.

- Reduce the amount of processed foods you eat and choose fresh whole foods instead such as fruits, vegetables, lean meats, fish, brown rice, potatoes, oats, whole grains, beans, lentils, fat-free dairy products, etc.

- When baking, replace some of the fat with applesauce or other pureed fruit. Use light or extra light olive oil for baking cakes or muffins.

- Try using low-fat yogurt to replace sour cream in recipes or baking.

- Replace one egg with two eggs whites in recipes to cut back on fat and cholesterol when possible.

The Carbohydrate Connection

Carbohydrates, or "carbs" as they are more commonly known, provide fuel for our body in the form of glucose (blood sugar) once they are broken down. They are found mainly in fruits, vegetables (especially starchy vegetables), dairy products, beans, and grains, including breads, cereals, rice, and pastas. The types of carbohydrates you choose or don't choose can have a direct impact on inflammation. There are three main types of carbohydrates in food:

- **Starches** (also called, "complex carbohydrates") include foods such as starchy vegetables like peas, corn, and potatoes; dried beans and lentils; grains (both refined and whole grains) such as breads, pasta, rice, oats, and barley. Starches are single sugars that are bonded together.

- **Sugars** (also called "simple carbohydrates") come in two main categories: naturally occurring such as the sugar found in fruits, milk, and other dairy products, and added sugars such as those added during processing including cookies, pastries, some cereals, and the list goes on. There are many different names for simple sugars including table sugar, honey, cane sugar, molasses, syrup, high fructose corn syrup, powdered sugar, beet sugar, and brown sugar. Sometimes you will find sugar listed by its chemical name such as sucrose or fructose. You can recognize other chemical names for sugar as they all end in "ose."

- **Fiber**, also considered a carbohydrate, comes strictly from plant foods and is the indigestible part of these foods. Good sources of fiber include foods such as whole grains, fruits, vegetables, beans, and nuts.

Whole Grains Versus Refined Grains

Whole grains include the entire grain kernel—bran, germ, and endosperm. The bran defines the outer layer of the grain and supplies antioxidants, B vitamins, trace minerals, and fiber. The germ is tiny but packs a powerful punch, supplying B vitamins, vitamin E, trace minerals, antioxidants, phytochemicals, essential fats, and fiber. The endosperm, or the inner part of the grain kernel, contains most of the protein and starchy carbohydrates supplying only small amounts of vitamins and minerals with no fiber. Whole grains include foods such as oatmeal, brown rice, wild rice, popcorn, whole wheat flour, corn, barley, whole wheat breads, quinoa, bran, whole grain couscous, and whole grain pasta. Whole grains are full of nutritional value and fiber to help slow down the absorption of sugar into the bloodstream.

Refined grains, on the other hand, have been milled, which is a process that removes the bran and germ from the grain, leaving only the endosperm. When the bran and germ are stripped away, so is about 25 percent of a grain's protein along with most of its key nutrients, including fiber. The milling is done to provide the grain with a finer texture and improve the shelf life. Refined grains include foods such as white flour, white rice, white breads, sugary cereals, crackers, flour tortillas, and white pastas. Many refined grains are enriched, meaning they add back some of the nutrients lost after milling, such as B vitamins and iron. However, fiber is not one of them, so refined grains have a much lower fiber content and higher glycemic index, which means they will raise blood sugar much quicker than a whole grain.

Your Nutrition Solution Tidbit

When choosing whole grain foods, look for the word "whole" on the label or in the ingredients. If, for example, the label states "wheat" bread, it is not a whole grain but if it states "whole wheat" bread, then it is. Check out *http://wholegrainscouncil.org* for more information on whole grains.

The Carbohydrates Best for Reducing Inflammation

So which carbohydrates are best to combat inflammation? When it comes to most starches you can go two ways, refined grains or whole grains. The path you want to take for both better health and reduced inflammation is that of the whole grains. A study in the *Journal of Nutrition* concluded that the protectiveness of whole grain consumption in relation to its positive effect on both type 2 diabetes and heart disease may be due to the effect these grains have on inflammatory protein concentrations. It concluded that this reinforces the public health recommendations of consuming whole grains on a daily basis. The researchers also found that refined grain intakes had a definite pro-inflammatory effect. A diet high in grains, specifically refined grains as well as added sugars, causes glucose (blood sugar) to build up in the blood stream. The result of high blood sugar is the release of IL-6 and TNF alpha, both of which are pro-inflammatory messengers.

The confirmed answer to which carbohydrates are best in reducing inflammation is, hands down, whole grains and to eliminate as many refined grains and added sugars as possible. Consuming whole grains may help to specifically decrease inflammation that is associated with metabolic syndrome, diabetes, and heart disease. However, making whole grains a part of your everyday diet will not only help you reduce inflammation, it will help you improve your overall health as well. Chapter 3 will provide you with tips on easy ways to begin incorporating whole grains into your everyday diet.

Your Nutrition Solution Tidbit

Metabolic syndrome is a cluster of risk factors that occur together and include high blood pressure, high fasting blood sugar levels, low high density lipoprotein (HDL) or "good" cholesterol, elevated triglyceride levels, and an excess amount of body fat around the abdomen and waist area. These conditions together can greatly increase your risk of heart disease, stroke, and type 2 diabetes. Any one of these conditions can increase your risk of serious disease, but together your risk becomes greater.

How Does Fiber Fit In?

High fiber foods can be helpful for blood sugar control, which we know can have an anti-inflammatory effect. Foods high in fiber allow the gradual release of insulin, which results in smaller levels of glucose being stored in the blood at any one time. In addition, a 2012 study in *Kidney International* (as well as many others) has found that high dietary total fiber intake is associated with a lower risk of chronic inflammation.

Fiber is a type of complex carbohydrate that is found only in plants and is frequently referred to as "roughage." It is the indigestible part of plant foods. Unlike other carbohydrates, the body does not digest or absorb fiber entirely so it contributes very few calories. Because of this, fiber is not truly considered a nutrient. However, you can still find it listed on food nutrient labels to help you choose fiber-rich foods.

There are two types of dietary fiber: soluble fiber and insoluble fiber. Both types benefit the body in many ways from promoting regularity, to preventing constipation, to decreasing the risk for colon cancer as well as other types of cancers. In addition, fiber helps to lower LDL (bad) cholesterol levels, reduce the risk for heart disease, and regulate blood sugar levels, all of which are associated with chronic inflammation. As if that weren't enough, high fiber foods can also help you feel fuller longer after you eat, which in turn can help you from nibbling when you shouldn't. And let's face it, fewer calories usually means weight loss, and a healthy body weight means less chance of inflammation.

Even though fiber isn't truly considered a nutrient, it is still a very important part of a healthy and well-balanced diet. Fiber can be found in loads of healthy foods including fruits, vegetables, legumes/beans, oatmeal, whole grains, soy foods, lentils, nuts, and seeds. How much fiber you need daily depends on your gender and age. As long as you stick close to the recommended servings of fruits, veggies, and whole grains, and often throw in some legumes/beans, nuts, and seeds, you should be able to meet your requirements. You will find more information about how to add more fiber to your diet in Chapter 3.

Supporting Nutrients

Research is uncovering pertinent information about how diet can play a major role in helping to reduce and/or eliminate chronic inflammation. Certain key vitamins and minerals may help to control the inflammatory processes in the body. Of course, it is vital to eat a healthy well-balanced diet to get all of the essential nutrients you need each day. However, some nutrients are more helpful than others when it comes to reducing inflammation.

Vitamin D

Vitamin D is essential to working with calcium to help strengthen bones and, in addition, it may also help protect against chronic inflammation. A deficiency of vitamin D has been associated with numerous inflammatory diseases including rheumatoid arthritis, IBD, certain types of cancer, and lupus. We can get vitamin D from foods, supplements, and even the sun. Vitamin D can be found in egg yolks, beef, liver, fish, and some fortified foods. Vitamin D is also produced within our body when our skin is exposed to sunlight. Vitamin D supplementation may help to reduce inflammation associated with age-related diseases. Taking a vitamin D supplement will not guarantee the prevention of these conditions nor has it been proven without a doubt that it will reduce inflammation in people with these types of conditions. However, experts feel that low levels of vitamin D are associated with high inflammatory markers, so your best bet is to ensure you get enough in your diet. If you don't feel you get enough sunlight or foods that include vitamin D, be sure to take a multivitamin that includes vitamin D. If you are still questionable about your intake, speak with your doctor about having a blood test to check your levels. If you plan to take a separate vitamin D supplement, speak with your doctor about dosage.

Your Nutrition Solution Tidbit

The Recommended Daily Allowance (RDA) for vitamin D for people 1 to 70 years of age, as well as pregnant and lactating women, is 600 IU (international units). The RDA jumps to 800 IU for those over 70 years old.

Vitamin C

Most of us think of vitamin C, or ascorbic acid, as protection against the common cold, but this water-soluble vitamin does much more than that. In addition to strengthening our immune system, vitamin C helps to produce collagen, which is the building block of the skin, as well as cartilage, ligaments in the joints, and blood vessels. It helps to heal wounds and form scar tissue. Adequate vitamin C intake is important to inflammation because it acts as an antioxidant and free radicals have a pro-inflammatory effect. Antioxidants help to rid the body of these inflammation-causing free radicals. In addition, taking vitamin C supplements may help to lower levels of CRP and other common inflammatory markers. One more benefit: vitamin C may also help to reduce tissue damage at inflammation sites. Vitamin C can be found in most fruits and vegetables, especially citrus fruits, and some fortified cereals and beverages. Most adults can get plenty of vitamin C if they eat at least five servings of fruits and vegetables daily.

Your Nutrition Solution Tidbit

The RDA for vitamin C is 90 mg for men 19 years and older and 75 mg for women 19 years and older. Some experts believe the RDA should be higher, around 200 mg, especially for the anti-inflammatory properties of vitamin C to be effective.

Vitamin E

Vitamin E is a fat-soluble vitamin with strong antioxidant properties that help protect essential fatty acids and vitamin A. Vitamin E helps to prevent cell damage and protect against free radicals, which may help to lower the risk for heart disease, stroke, cancer, and other diseases of aging. In addition, vitamin E aids in the formation and functioning of red blood cells and other tissues. Vitamin E has effects on the inflammatory process because of the antioxidant functions of alpha-tocopherol, a powerful form of vitamin E. Alpha-tocopherol is believed to decrease CRP levels as well as pro-inflammatory markers including cytokines. Vitamin E can be found in vegetable oils, nuts, seeds, whole grains, wheat germ, fortified cereals and foods, green leafy vegetables, and olives. Experts have found that the typical diet of most Americans, especially those on a low-fat diet, may provide less than the RDA levels for vitamin E, so it is important to be aware of the foods that contain vitamin E and to speak with your doctor if you feel you are not getting enough. Always discuss with your doctor before taking a separate supplement.

Your Nutrition Solution Tidbit

The RDA for vitamin E is 15 mg (22.4 IU) for both males and females over the age of 14 years.

Vitamin B6

Vitamin B6 is a member of the B vitamin family and is a water-soluble vitamin. This vitamin is responsible for non-essential amino acids, which in turn are used to make body cells. It aids in the formation of insulin, red blood cells, and antibodies in addition to maintaining normal brain function. Because vitamin B6 is a water-soluble vitamin, it does not get stored in the body so you need to restock it daily through foods you consume. Vitamin B6 can be found in lean meats and poultry, legumes, whole grain cereals, whole grain flour, wheat germ, fish and seafood, lentils, green leafy vegetables, other vegetables, bananas, potatoes, milk, cheese, and eggs. Not getting enough vitamin B6 can increase levels of CRP, a marker for inflammation that has been linked to heart disease. In addition, a lack of B6 can possibly increase inflammation that is associated with rheumatoid arthritis.

Your Nutrition Solution Tidbit

The RDA for vitamin B6 is 1.3 milligrams (mg) for adults 19 to 50 years of age. Over 50 years of age, men need 1.7 mg and women need 1.5 mg. Taking too much B6 through supplementation can cause nerve damage. Speak with your doctor before taking an additional supplement.

Zinc

Zinc is an essential mineral that is required for the catalytic activity of nearly 100 enzymes in our body. It plays a major role in immune function, protein synthesis, wound healing, DNA synthesis, and cell division. In addition, zinc supports normal growth and development during pregnancy, childhood, and adolescence and is needed for our senses of taste and smell. On top of all of that, researchers have found that zinc may have some benefits in the reduction of inflammation. A study published in the January 2013 *Journal of Nutritional Biochemistry* suggested that restoring zinc status via a dietary supplement reduced age-associated inflammation. It seems that zinc deficiency has been found in a number of diseases associated with inflammation such as rheumatoid arthritis, type 2 diabetes, and certain cancers. Findings in this and other studies have concluded that zinc may have a protective effect in certain health issues because of its anti-inflammatory and antioxidant functions.

It is first important to ensure you are getting plenty of zinc in your diet through foods and are not deficient before starting supplements. Never start any type of supplement before speaking with your doctor, as there are usually precautions when taking supplements of single nutrients and there can be issues if taken too much. High doses of zinc in supplement form can actually decrease immune levels, interfere with copper absorption, and increase the risk for anemia. Zinc can be found in a large variety of foods, including oysters, beef, crab, eggs, fortified breakfast cereals, pork, legumes, dark meat chicken, yogurt, nuts, pumpkin seeds, chickpeas, and oatmeal and other whole grains.

Your Nutrition Solution Tidbit

The RDA for zinc for adult males (19 years and older) is 11 mg per day and 8 mg for females. Amounts are slightly higher for pregnant and lactating women. Speak with your doctor about supplementation if you feel you may be deficient and are not getting enough zinc through your diet.

Magnesium

Magnesium is a mineral that can be found in the body in our bones, teeth, and red blood cells. It is essential for the proper functioning of the nervous, muscular, and cardiovascular systems. A diet that is rich in magnesium can help to lower your risk for metabolic syndrome and its risk factors. In addition, this mineral helps to promote normal blood pressure, helps keep the heart rhythm steady, and is also involved in the energy metabolism pathway. This essential nutrient is one that a good majority of Americans do not get enough of, with a typical intake below the RDA. Adults that do not consume enough magnesium are more likely to have increased inflammation markers. Good dietary sources of magnesium include whole grains, green leafy vegetables (such as spinach), almonds and other nuts, avocados, beans, and soybeans. A diet that is high in fat, as many Americans' are, can cause less magnesium to be absorbed—another good case for a lower-fat diet.

Your Nutrition Solution Tidbit

The RDA for magnesium for adult males 19 to 30 years of age is 400 mg; for 31 years and older, it's 420 mg. For adult females 19 to 30 years, the RDA is 310 mg; for 31 years and older, it's 320 mg. It is slightly higher for pregnant and lactating women. Taking too much magnesium in the form of supplements can have ill effects and even be toxic if taken in extreme high doses. Magnesium supplements can also interact with some medications, so speak with your doctor about safety and dosage if you are thinking of taking a magnesium supplement.

Polyphenol Antioxidants

Polyphenols are the most abundant antioxidants in the diet and can be found in a large variety of fruits, vegetables, whole grains, chocolate, coffee, olive oil, flaxseed, tea, and more. Thousands of these compounds have been identified and classified into two major groups: flavonoids and lignans. Polyphenols play a role in the prevention of degenerative diseases, especially cardiovascular diseases and certain cancers. In addition, these powerful compounds show a powerful anti-inflammatory effect by decreasing pro-inflammatory cytokine production and helping to block the activity of pro-inflammatory signaling systems. Ongoing studies of polyphenols continue because there is such a wide variety of these compounds and their content in foods varies so greatly. There is much more to find out, so for now be sure to include some of these healthy foods that contain polyphenols as it may add some anti-inflammatory benefits.

Discovering Supplements

Supplements can be another avenue to explore when trying to manage inflammation. There are both pros and cons when dealing with supplements. For some, they can be an effective and more natural means to treating pain and other symptoms caused by chronic inflammation and can sometimes take the place of OTC and prescription medications, or at the least help to minimize usage of both. On the other hand, dietary supplements are not regulated by the Food and Drug Administration (FDA) as prescription drugs are, so their safety and proven effectiveness can sometimes be questionable. However, it is important to point out that natural and prescription pain relievers and inflammation reducers don't need to stand in opposition. There are times when they can be used together as a powerful tool. Always see your doctor first before starting any type of OTC dietary or herbal supplement, especially if you are currently taking prescription medications. Never stop a prescription medication and replace it with any type of supplement without speaking with your doctor first.

Dietary Supplements

A dietary supplement is defined by the Dietary Supplement Health and Education Act (DSHEA) as a product that:

- Is intended to supplement the diet.
- Contains one or more dietary ingredients (including vitamins, minerals, herbs, or other botanicals,

amino acids, and certain other substances) or their constituents.

- Is intended to be taken by mouth, in forms such as tablet, capsule, powder, softgel, gelcap, or liquid.
- Is labeled as being a dietary supplement.

Your Nutrition Solution Tidbit

According to NCCAM (the National Center for Complementary and Alternative Medicine), the DSHEA is a federal law that defines dietary supplements and sets product-labeling standards and health claim limits. DSHEA defines supplements and outlines quality, safety, and efficacy regulations that are different from those for drugs.

Probiotics

The World Health Organization (WHO) defines probiotics as "live microorganisms, which when administered in adequate amounts, confer a health benefit to the host." Probiotics are often referred to as "good bacteria" and are available in products such as dietary supplements and yogurts. The FDA has not yet approved any health claims for probiotics to date. The idea behind probiotics is that our lower gastrointestinal tract, or our "gut," contains a whole community of complex and various bacteria. Although the word bacteria tends to conjure up thoughts of harmful germs, many bacteria are actually helpful and essential to the body for proper and peak performance and are commonly known as "good bacteria." Most probiotics are very similar to these good bacteria that are found naturally in our gut. Many of the probiotics used in the United States include two major groups called *Lactobacillus* and *Bifidobacterium*.

What does this all have to do with inflammation? The beneficial bacteria found in yogurt and probiotic supplements tend to keep in check the "bad" bacteria that also live in our gut and generate an anti-inflammatory response. Much research continues on probiotics as scientists uncover more and more about their potential health benefits. Probiotic supplements may contain different types of probiotic bacteria depending on the product and what it is intended for. Check with your doctor before choosing a probiotic and do not use it to replace any prescription medication without first speaking with your doctor.

Your Nutrition Solution Tidbit

When choosing yogurt, look for the words "live active cultures" to be sure the yogurt you select has the probiotics you expect.

GLA (Gamma-Linolenic Acid)

Gamma-linolenic acid (GLA) is an omega-6 fatty acid. Those might sound familiar as we already talked about them earlier in this chapter. GLA is found mostly in plant-based oils such as borage seed oil, evening primrose oil, and black currant seed oil. Many omega-6 fatty acids in the diet come from vegetable oils in the form of linoleic acid (LA). The body converts linoleic acid to GLA and then to arachidonic acid (AA). Linoleic acid and arachidonic acid tend to be unhealthy and promote inflammation. On the other hand, GLA tends to actually help reduce inflammation. Much of the GLA that is taken in the form of a supplement is converted to something called

DGLA (Dihomo-gamma-linolenic acid) that helps to reduce inflammation. Having enough of certain nutrients in the body such as magnesium, zinc, vitamin C, and vitamin B6 helps to promote the conversion of GLA to DGLA. Having too much AA in our body can prevent LA from converting into GLA. It is when we have too much LA in the body that a problem can arise as it causes an imbalance between pro-inflammatory and anti-inflammatory nutrients. When we consume more anti-inflammatory nutrients such as GLA, we can help balance out the equation. Most GLA supplements come in the form of oil-containing capsules.

Your Nutrition Solution Tidbit

GLA supplements in doses higher than 3,000 mg per day can actually backfire and increase inflammation in the body. How much is recommended daily depends on many individual factors including the condition you are being treated for, age, weight, and medications and/or supplements being used. GLA can negatively interact with certain prescription medications as well as other supplements, so speak with your doctor before starting a GLA supplement.

Herbal Supplements

There are countless herbal supplements on the market with many being useful for treating the symptoms of inflammation and/or helping to reduce inflammation. If you are open to trying a more natural approach and would like to add herbal supplements to your treatment plan of diet, lifestyle, and possible prescription medication, speak with your doctor first about safety and dosage. Herbal supplements, although natural, can trigger side effects, and can interact with other herbs, supplements, and medications (both OTC and prescription). You should use precautions when taking herbs and do so under the supervision of your doctor only. Following are some of the more common herbal supplements that can have a positive effect on inflammation and its symptoms.

Zyflamend

Zyflamend is a dietary supplement that contains 10 different herbs and is marketed for a healthy inflammation response as well as for normal cardiovascular and joint function. Preliminary studies have shown that the combination of ingredients in Zyflamend have anti-inflammatory properties by helping to suppress elevated levels of pro-inflammatory markers. The ingredients in Zyflamend are holy basil, turmeric, ginger, green tea, rosemary, Hu Zhang (a rich source of resveratrol), Chinese goldthread, barberry, oregano, and skullcap.

Pycnogenol

Pycnogenol is another dietary supplement touted as an anti-inflammatory. It is obtained from the bark of the French maritime pine tree as an extract. This supplement has been found to have not only anti-inflammatory properties but also antioxidant, immunostimulant, and neuro-protective effects, as well as antiviral and antimicrobial activity. Pycnogenol can interact with other medications.

Cat's Claw

Cat's claw, or *Uncaria tomentosa*, has indicated modest benefits for easing the joint pain caused by rheumatoid arthritis and osteoarthritis knee pain by reducing inflammation. Evidence does not show that it prevents joint damage from persisting. Further studies are being done for other possible uses with other health conditions associated with inflammation such as lupus, Crohn's disease, and Alzheimer's, for example. Cat's claw can be used in the form of teas, capsules, or extracts.

Devil's Claw

Devil's claw, or *Harpagophytum procumbens*, is used to treat rheumatoid arthritis as well as soothe pain resulting from osteoarthritis, tendonitis, back/muscle pain, and neck troubles. This herb is also used commonly as an anti-inflammatory agent.

Willow Bark

Willow bark is made from several varieties of willow trees in which the bark is used to make the herbal supplement. Willow bark mirrors the same effects of aspirin and tends to be used to reduce pain and inflammation from rheumatoid arthritis, osteoarthritis, gout, muscle pain, and headaches. Willow bark is available as a powdered herb, dried herb, or tincture.

Slippery Elm

Slippery elm, or *Ulmus fulva*, has been used for centuries and comes from the inner bark of the Slippery Elm tree. This herb contains antioxidants that help to relieve inflammatory bowel conditions. In addition, it is often suggested for other inflammatory conditions such as Crohn's disease, ulcerative colitis, and irritable bowel syndrome (IBS). Slippery elm is available in tablets, capsules, lozenges, teas, and extracts. You should take slippery elm two hours before or after taking any other herbs or medications.

Saw Palmetto

Saw palmetto, or *Serenoa repens*, is a type of slow growing palm tree that is native to the southeastern part of the United States. The ripe fruit of the tree is rich in fatty acids and phytosterols, which have been used to help reduce inflammation. The fruit is used in several forms including ground and dried fruit and whole berries. Saw palmetto is available as a liquid extract, tablets, capsules, and as tea.

Boswellia

Boswellia, or *boswellia serrata*, contains boswellic acids that in animal studies have shown to significantly reduce inflammation and have anti-arthritic effects. It is normally available in capsule form.

chapter 3

your 5-step nutrition and lifestyle solution

What we put in our bodies nutritionally and how we treat our bodies physically can have a huge impact on our overall health, including inflammation. This chapter will go into detail on five steps you can start following now to help eliminate, prevent, and/or reduce chronic inflammation. Nutrition and lifestyle changes will help you to feel better as well as lower your risk for many chronic diseases. The key is to be hands-on and to make lifestyle changes that will be permanent and help remedy your problems long term. All five of these steps are matters you *do* have control over. Focus on your personalized objectives and set achievable goals for yourself. That is the secret to making lasting dietary and lifestyle changes that will combat inflammation and enhance your overall health. Now is the time to empower yourself and take action!

Step 1. Go Mediterranean!

When it comes to the typical American diet, a red flag warning for chronic inflammation is front and center. Unfortunately, the typical diet of most Americans is a major culprit when it comes to the health conditions associated with chronic inflammation. All types of diets have been deemed "the" anti-inflammatory diet. A 2006 study published in the *Journal of the American College of Cardiology* found that diets that are high in refined starches, added sugars, saturated fats, and trans fats as well as low in fruits, vegetables, whole grains, and omega-3 fatty acids appear to trigger the inflammatory response. But on the other hand, a diet rich in whole unprocessed foods, healthy fats, lean protein sources, whole grains, and loads of fruits and vegetables, along with regular exercise seems to calm down the inflammation response.

As luck would have it, there is a diet out there that covers just about all of those bases. That diet would be the Mediterranean diet, which many experts recommend when it comes to an anti-inflammatory diet or way of eating. The Mediterranean diet isn't really a "diet" in the sense that we are used to, meaning it isn't a typical weight-loss plan, but instead a healthy and lifelong change to eating and lifestyle. The Mediterranean diet is about a total eating plan and less about any one single food that generates healthy benefits and longevity. It revolves around how particular healthy cuisine from all of the food groups and a healthier lifestyle work cohesively to construct the diet and make it what it is. This style of eating is associated with countries that surround the Mediterranean sea, mostly Spain, Italy, and Greece. Although many of the authentic foods that are native to these areas may seem difficult to follow, you can still "Americanize" it and have it remain heart healthy and anti-inflammatory.

Mediterranean Diet Benefits

The Mediterranean diet is known to help lower the risk of heart disease and improve cardiovascular health, raise HDL (good cholesterol) and lower LDL (bad cholesterol), aide in weight management, protect against certain types of cancers, and ward off depression. It can also manage type 2 diabetes, lower the risk for hypertension, decrease the risk for mental decline and Alzheimer's disease, help protect against Parkinson's disease, and last but not least, help reduce inflammation in rheumatoid arthritis. Many of these are inflammatory-related diseases and health conditions, so it makes sense that following this type of eating style would help decrease or eliminate the inflammation response.

What It's All About

The Mediterranean diet is not a tough one to follow and much easier to incorporate into your daily life than you may think. In fact, much of it is about basically eating a healthy diet. The key components of the Mediterranean diet include:

- Minimal intake of processed, refined, and low-nutrient foods and incorporating more whole foods.

- Generous amounts of fresh fruits and vegetables that are preferably locally grown.

- Increase in plant foods as opposed to animal foods, including legumes (dried beans), soy foods, whole grains, nuts and seeds, as well as fruits and vegetables.

- Whole grains such as pastas, cereals, breads, and other grain products that are high in fiber and have a low glycemic index. (I will explain glycemic index later in the chapter.)

- Moderate amounts of fish (especially fatty fish) and shellfish with low to moderate amounts of poultry, eggs, and other lean meats to help meet protein needs. Red meats are used very little, if at all.

- Moderate amounts of dairy products that are fat-free or at least low-fat.

- Healthy fats, not just from fish and foods such as avocados and nuts, but also from the use of mono-unsaturated fats, especially olive oil. Butter, margarine, and other fats containing saturated or trans fats are avoided.

- Herbs and spices to flavor foods instead of using salt.

- Sugars that come from natural sources such as fruit and honey.

- Small amounts of red wine mostly with meals, in moderation of course. (If you don't drink, don't start. You can always use purple grape juice as an alternative.)

The Mediterranean diet also promotes staying active and balancing calories to promote an optimal and healthy weight. Compared with the typical American diet, the Mediterranean diet is rich in fiber, polyphenols, antioxidants, phytonutrients, monounsaturated fats, and omega-3 fatty acids, all of which have a positive impact on inflammation. In addition, it has a much healthier balance between omega-3 and omega-6 fatty acids. Clinical studies have demonstrated that consuming a Mediterranean style diet helps to reduce plasma levels of pro-inflammatory markers including CRP, TNF-alpha, and others.

Adopting This Eating Style

Now that you are aware of the key components of this diet, it's time to start making some changes. Don't try to change everything all in one day. Your goal should be to approach needed changes step by step and adapt to this new way of eating a little at a time. Trying to make changes all at once can be very overwhelming and often can lead to the demise of your best intentions. The most important concept is to make new changes consistently while continuing the ones you have already made. If it seems overwhelming, try writing down your goals weekly to keep track of your success.

Tips for Shifting to the Mediterranean Diet

- Substitute or replace foods in moderation. You don't want to jump in all at once, especially if your diet needs a lot of help.

- Start using extra virgin olive oil or canola oil as your main fat source instead of less healthy fats such as margarine or butter. Use it in cooking as well as in place of your favorite salad dressing or on bread for items such as garlic toast. Keep in mind that even healthy fats contain lots of calories, so eat them in moderation and watch portion sizes.

- Visualize your plate (watch plate size and use a smaller-sized one to control calories and portions) in a different way and fill at least half of it with fruits and vegetables. Fill the other side with mostly whole grains and the rest with a small amount of protein in the form of fish, nuts, beans, lentils, and lean white meats. This is much like the ChooseMyPlate icon from the United States Department of Agriculture (USDA) that you can find out more about at *www.choosemyplate.gov.*

- Use snack-time wisely and treat it as a chance to consume more fruits, vegetables, nuts, and seeds.

- Visit your local produce markets to buy produce or maybe even start your own garden!

- Introduce a new fruit and vegetable each week to your meal plans. Don't be afraid to experiment with new foods. You can use fresh or frozen produce and be sure to include a variety for a better nutritional intake.

- When creating your weekly meal plans, substitute grilled, broiled, or steamed fatty fish, such as salmon, sardines, tuna, mackerel, and trout, instead of red meat or other high-fat meats at least two times per week. Each week reduce the amount of red and/or high fat meats you eat as well as the portion sizes.

- Switch refined grains such as white bread, white rice, or white pasta for whole grains such as whole wheat bread, brown rice, and whole wheat pasta.

- Try out whole grains of the Mediterranean such as barley, bulgur, and couscous by using some new recipes.

- Plan a few meatless meals each week and make legumes or beans the main focus of those meals.

- Switch to soft cheese that is naturally low in fat, fat-free milk, and fat-free or low-fat plain yogurt; Greek yogurt is a better choice because it is higher in protein.

- Season your foods and recipes with herbs and spices instead of salt. It may take some practice and experimentation to get good at it! Chapter 4 will discuss some herbs and spices that are beneficial for inflammation.

- Cook more of your meals from scratch, cutting back on the amount of processed foods you eat daily. Invest in a few good Mediterranean and healthy cookbooks to help get you started and get those creative juices flowing.

- Instead of sweets, baked goods, and other fat- and sugar-laden desserts and treats, replace them with fresh fruit, fruit desserts, and nuts.

- If approved by your doctor, try adding a glass of red wine at dinner. If you don't drink, try substituting purple grape juice to reap some of the health benefits.

Your Nutrition Solution Tidbit

Red wine is a staple in the Mediterranean and the heart-healthy benefits of it come from an antioxidant known as polyphenols with one called resveratrol found specifically in red wine. Research shows that resveratrol might be linked to a reduced risk of inflammation and blood clotting, which in turn can lower the risk for heart disease. The resveratrol in red wine comes from the skin of the grapes used to make the wine. Because red wine is fermented with grape skins longer than that of white wine, the red varieties contain much more resveratrol. You can also eat red or purple grapes or drink 100 percent grape juice for some of the benefits as well. Other foods that contain resveratrol include peanuts, blueberries, and cranberries. However, if you don't drink alcohol, don't start. And if you want to add red wine occasionally, ask your doctor first. You can also get resveratrol in a supplement form. The resveratrol in these supplements, though, comes not from the skin of red grape but from the Japanese knotweed plant.

These are all simple suggestions to help get you started. And remember that you don't have to tackle them all at the same time. You will read many tips and helpful hints throughout this book that should assist you in transitioning your diet. Some you will hear more than once, but that is because of their importance. Once you begin to incorporate some of these suggestions into your daily life, you will begin to realize how simple, healthy, and tasty eating an anti-inflammatory diet can be.

Your Nutrition Solution Tidbit

If you are interested in finding out more about the Mediterranean diet, check out *The Complete Idiot's Guide to The Mediterranean Diet* (Alpha Books, 2010).

Clean Eating

Another popular and anti-inflammatory eating style is the "Clean Eating" diet. It has many of the same elements as the Mediterranean diet and can be another way to ward off inflammation. The basis of the Clean Eating diet that we hear so much about lately is consuming foods in their most natural state, or as close to it as possible. Much like the Mediterranean diet, the Clean Eating diet is not a "diet" but a lifestyle approach to food and the way it is prepared, leading to better health. Combining this type of lifestyle approach with the elements of the Mediterranean diet and choosing the foods within your diet that are anti-inflammatory can have a big impact on your overall health, chronic inflammation, energy levels, and the basic way you feel every day.

Here are some of the main points of the Clean Eating diet (you may notice that many of them sound familiar as points we have already recommended in this book):

- **Eat five to six times per day.** Eat three moderate meals and two to three small snacks each day, eating every two to three hours. Include lean protein, fresh fruits and vegetables, and a complex carbohydrate, especially whole grains with each meal. This helps to keep your body fueled and burning calories efficiently all day long. It also gives you more opportunities to include the foods you need daily, especially fruits and veggies.

- **Drink at least eight cups of water daily.** Water is not only essential for the proper functioning of the body, but it can help with metabolism, energy levels, lubricating sore joints, appetite, and so much more.

- **Get label savvy.** "Clean" foods should contain no more than one to two ingredients. Any food product with a long list of ingredients, especially ones you have never heard of, are not considered clean.

- **Avoid processed and refined foods.** These foods include any product made with white flour and sugar such as breads, pasta, etc. Choose complex carbohydrates such as whole grains instead.

- **Know the enemies.** Avoid all foods high in saturated and trans fats, fried foods, and anything high in refined sugar.

- **Choose the right meat.** It is recommended to choose grass-fed or local meats.

- **Whenever possible, go organic.** Choose organic produce and other foods as often as possible. If budget restraints don't allow this, make meat, eggs, dairy, and "the dirty dozen" fruits and vegetables your priority.

- **Consume healthy fats.** Include essential fatty acids, especially omega-3 fatty acids daily.

- **Be aware of portion sizes.** Work toward eating within moderate portions.

- **Reduce your carbon footprint.** Strive to eat produce that is seasonal and locally grown.

- **Slow down and enjoy.** Don't rush through your meals. Slow down and savor the taste of clean foods and enjoy every bite.

- **Take it to go.** Pack your cooler for work lunches, outings, etc. so that you are always prepared and have clean food when you are out and about.

- **Get the family involved.** Don't just do this for yourself; make it a family affair. Improve the quality of your family's life and health along with yours.

Your Nutrition Solution Tidbit

The Environmental Working Group has put together 12 fruits and vegetables that are the most contaminated with the highest pesticide residue. If you are not up for buying everything organic, they suggest at least buying the following in organic form:

- Peaches.
- Apples.
- Sweet bell pepper.
- Celery.

- Nectarines.
- Strawberries.
- Cherries.
- Pears.
- Grapes (imported).
- Spinach.
- Potatoes.
- Lettuce.

They recommend the following 12 fruits and vegetables as the least contaminated:

- Onions.
- Avocado.
- Sweet corn (frozen).
- Pineapple.
- Mango.
- Asparagus.
- Sweet peas (frozen).
- Kiwi fruit.
- Bananas.
- Cabbage.
- Broccoli.
- Papaya.

For more information check out: *www.ewg.org.*

Step 2. Be Choosey About Carbohydrates

As we learned in Chapter 2, there is more than one way to look at a carbohydrate and the type you choose can mean the difference between inflammation and little to no inflammation. Keep in mind that carbohydrates encompass starches, sugar, and fiber.

Swap Whole Grains for Refined Grains

We discussed in Chapter 2 why choosing whole grains over refined grains is so important for reduction of inflammation. Whole grains are much healthier and offer much more in the way of nutritional value than refined grains do. Refined grains have been shown to possess pro-inflammatory markers, so the more we swap those refined grains for whole grains the better. Refined grains include a lot of the foods Americans typically eat, such as white breads, tortillas, pizza crust, white rice, pasta, cookies, cakes, donuts, and other desserts, just to name a few. Swapping these foods for whole grains is a small change that can make a big difference in both managing your symptoms of inflammation as well as helping to eliminate and prevent chronic inflammation. Whole grains include whole wheat breads, brown rice, wild rice, popcorn, whole grain pasta, whole grain couscous, barley, oats, bulgur, and corn, for instance. Upping your whole grain intake as well as decreasing your refined grain intake are both part of the Mediterranean style of eating as well as part of the U.S. Dietary Guidelines for Americans. The current Dietary Guidelines for Americans recommends that all adults eat at least half of their grains as whole grains. That adds up to at least three to five servings of whole grains daily. Examples of *one* serving include:

- 1 slice bread.
- 1 cup ready-to-eat cereal.
- 1/2 cup oatmeal.
- 1/2 cup rice.
- 1/2 English muffin.

- 3 cups popcorn.
- 1/2 cup pasta.

Your Nutrition Solution Tidbit

ChooseMyPlate.gov and the Dietary Guidelines for Americans are issued and updated jointly by the Department of Agriculture (USDA) and the Department of Health and Human Services (HHS) every five years. Both guidelines work hand-in-hand to provide the most current scientific-based advice for all Americans two years old and older. They are available for all Americans so that we can educate ourselves as to what good nutrition is and how we can make healthier choices. The newest set of Dietary Guidelines for Americans focuses on three major goals that together emphasize a total lifestyle approach:

1. Balancing calories with physical activity to manage weight.

2. Consuming more healthy foods and nutrients such as fruits, vegetables, whole grains, fat-free and low-fat dairy products, and seafood.

3. Consuming fewer foods with sodium (salt), saturated fats, trans fats, cholesterol, added sugars, and refined grains.

For more information, you are encouraged to check out: *www.choosemyplate.gov/* and *www.cnpp.usda.gov/DietaryGuidelines*.

Tips for Switching to Whole Grains

Not sure where to get started? Here are a few tips to help you out:

- Try rolled oats, steel-cut oats, barley, buckwheat, or other whole grains as a hot breakfast cereal in place of white toast or sugary cereals.

- Substitute half of the refined flour for whole wheat flour in your baked goods recipes. You can even try adding up to 20 percent of another whole grain flour such as sorghum. You can also use whole grain flour as a thickener when a recipe calls for it.

- Step up your breakfast foods by making pancakes or muffins using a combination of whole grain flours instead of refined white flour.

- Choose whole grain bread, buns, rolls, pita, English muffins, and bagels in place of ones made with refined white flour. Check the label for the word "whole" so you know you are getting an actual whole grain product.

- Switch your sugary breakfast cereal to one that contains whole grains, more fiber, and less sugar.

- Try brown rice or wild rice as a side dish or in a casserole in place of white rice. Instead of rice, you can even try whole grain couscous, barley, or bulgur as well.

- Buy whole grain pasta or one that is a blend of whole grain and white pasta instead of refined white pasta. Use them with your favorite sauces or in casseroles, soups, and salads.

- Add cooked bulgur, brown or wild rice, whole grain couscous, or barley to your favorite canned or homemade soup for an instant serving or more of whole grains.

- Jazz up your holiday bread stuffing with cooked bulgur, wild rice, or barley.

- Add three-quarters of a cup of uncooked oats to each pound of ground turkey or chicken breast to make meatballs, stuffed peppers, burgers, or meatloaf. Add whole grains to and make a great meat extender.

- Stir in a handful of rolled oats to your low-fat yogurt.

- Use oat bran to coat fish or chicken in place of refined bread crumbs.

- Look for snack foods, such as chips, that are made with whole grains instead of your go-to potato chips.

- Check out new recipes from sources such as the Whole Grains Council to sharpen your whole grain cooking skills (see: *http://wholegrainscouncil.org/*).

How to Find Whole Grains

You want to switch to eating more whole grains and weeding out the refined grains, but how do you know what foods are and are not made with whole grains? The "Whole Grain Stamp" from the Whole Grains Council makes it easier than you think. There are actually two different stamps that show up on packaged foods:

- **100% Stamp:** means that all of the grains in the product are whole grains and that there is a minimum of 18 grams (a full serving) of whole grains per labeled serving.

- **Basic Stamp:** means it contains at least 10 grams (a half serving) of whole grains per labeled serving, but the product may also contain some refined grain. Even if a product contains larger amounts of whole grains, it will use the Basic Stamp if it contains any refined grain product.

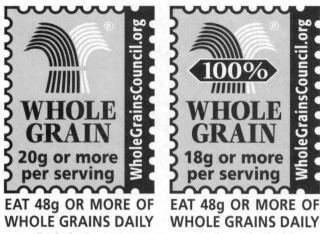

"Whole Grain Stamps® are a trademark of Oldways Preservation Trust and the Whole Grains Council, www. wholegrainscouncil.org. Used with permission.

Because the Whole Grain Stamp is not yet on all packaged foods, you still need to be aware of what to look for on labels. If there is no stamp, you can look for wording on the label that might state something like "100% whole wheat," which is a statement you can trust. But if you see something like "whole grain" without a little more explanation, you might need to investigate further. That can mean that the food only contains a very tiny amount of whole grains. You should check the ingredient list. If the first ingredient listed contains the word "whole" such as "whole wheat flour," then it's likely the food is mostly whole grains. If there are two flours listed and only the second one states "whole," the product could contain anywhere from 1 to 49 percent whole grains.

The following words on a label would mean that you are getting a whole grain:

- Whole grain, whole wheat, whole (other grain).
- Stone-ground whole (grain).
- Brown rice.
- Wheat berries.
- Oats, oatmeal.

The following words on a label would mean that the food is most likely missing some part of the whole grain:

- Wheat or wheat flour.
- Semolina.
- Durum wheat.
- Organic flour.
- Stone-ground.
- Multigrain.

The following words on a label would definitely mean the food is not a whole grain:

- Enriched flour.
- De-germinated corn meal.
- Bran.
- Wheat germ.

Your Nutrition Solution Tidbit

Fiber content can vary from grain to grain and is not a good predictor of whole grain content.

The key is to begin finding ways to fit whole grains in anywhere you can. Remember that a little bit can go a long way, but shoot for as many as possible. Always check food labels and ingredient lists to ensure you are actually buying a whole grain product. Continue to gather information about whole grains and the vast variety that is out there to try.

Discovering Glycemic Index and Glycemic Load

Choosing whole grains over refined grains is important because, as we learned in Chapter 2, a diet high in grains, specifically refined grains as well as added sugars, causes blood sugar spikes, which in turn causes glucose (blood sugar) to build up in the blood stream. The result of high blood sugar is the release of IL-6 and TNF alpha, both of which are pro-inflammatory messengers. Recommendations for reducing inflammation are not only to lower your consumption of refined grains, but to choose foods with a lower glycemic index. Most whole grains tend to have a lower glycemic index, but not all. Glycemic index (GI) measures how much and how quickly each gram of available carbohydrate (total carbohydrate minus the fiber) in a single food affects your blood sugar level. Glycemic index only pertains to foods that contain carbohydrates, so foods such as meat and fats do not have a GI. Foods are ranked with an "index" by how they compare to pure glucose that has a GI of 100 per 50 grams. A food with a high GI raises blood sugar higher and quicker, whereas a food with a medium or low GI does the opposite. Foods that tend to have a lower GI are those that contain fiber and fat. Both of these nutrients slow down the absorption of glucose into the blood stream. Other factors such as the ripeness of a fruit, processing, cooking method, and variety of a food can affect the GI.

Keep in mind that some very nutritious foods have a higher GI than some not so nutritious foods. Just because a food has a high or low glycemic index does not necessarily mean a food is "healthy" or not. However, sticking with lower GI foods and/or balancing meals with both can help to keep blood sugar levels from spiking and therefore keep glucose from building up in your blood stream and contributing to inflammation.

Examples of Low GI Foods (55 or Less)

- 100 percent stone-ground whole wheat bread.
- Pumpernickel bread.
- Corn/wheat tortilla.
- Brown rice.
- Oatmeal or oat bran.
- Legumes and lentils.
- Avocados.
- Apples.
- Hummus.
- Nuts.
- Milk.

Examples of Medium GI Foods (56–69)

- Sweet potato.
- Couscous.
- Banana.
- Grapes.
- White spaghetti noodles.
- White rice.

Examples of High GI Foods (70 or More)

- White breads.
- Baked goods.
- Crackers.
- White potatoes.
- Kiwi.
- Pineapple.
- Watermelon.

The glycemic load is based on the glycemic index. However, it takes into account not only the effect on blood sugar, but also the amount of carbohydrate in the food. Glycemic load is calculated by multiplying a foods glycemic index by the amount of carbohydrates it contains. Because the glycemic load includes both components, a specific food can have a high glycemic index but a low glycemic load, making it a better choice than it may have originally appeared. Using glycemic load can help to control blood sugar levels, which can be a helpful tool when trying to reduce chronic inflammation levels. Both glycemic index and glycemic load can be tough to figure out at first. If you are having problems, see an RDN for more explanation and instruction on how to incorporate it into your meal planning as a tool to reducing and eliminating chronic inflammation.

Examples of Low Glycemic Load (10 and Under)

- High fiber fruits and vegetables (excluding white potatoes).
- Bran cereals.
- Most dried beans, legumes, and lentils.
- Most nuts.
- Milk.

Examples of Low Medium Load (11–19)

- Brown rice.
- Oatmeal.
- Whole grain bread.
- Bulgur.
- Whole grain pasta.
- Sweet potato.

Examples of Low High Load (20 or More)

- White potato.
- French fries.
- Couscous.
- Refined (sugary) breakfast cereal.
- White breads.

Filling Up on Fiber

Switching from refined grains to whole grains and adding more plant foods such as fruits, vegetables, nuts, and seeds is a great way to fill up on fiber. We learned from Chapter 2 that a high fiber diet can actually help to lower our risk for inflammation. So how much do we actually need? The recommendations by the Institute of Medicine's Food and Nutrition Board state:

- Adult women under 50 years of age = 25 grams daily. (That amount increases during pregnancy and breastfeeding.)
- Adult women over 50 years of age = 21 grams daily.
- Adult men under 50 years of age = 38 grams daily.
- Adult men over 50 years of age = 30 grams daily.

Gastrointestinal side effects such as gas, constipation, indigestion, and cramping can be potential barriers to achieving a higher fiber intake. It is best to take it in small steps. Start by getting at least 14 grams per 1,000 calories. From there you can step up your intake gradually. Always drink plenty of water as you increase fiber intake as well. This can help alleviate some side effects and keep the fiber smoothly moving through the digestive tract.

Here are a few simple ways to increase your daily fiber:

- Start your day with a bowl of whole grain cereal, either hot or cold, and top it with sliced fresh fruit.
- Make the switch from white breads to whole grain breads, refined pasta to whole wheat pastas, and white rice to brown or wild rice. In other words, follow the previous tips about switching from refined grains to whole grains.
- Add barley, beans, lentils, and split peas to salads, soups, casseroles, and stews.
- Grab a piece of fresh fruit when you get that afternoon sweet tooth.
- Do not overcook vegetables. Instead, lightly steam them to keep the fiber intact.
- Sneak fiber into a sandwich with shredded carrots, sliced cucumbers, sliced tomato, raw spinach, and sprouts in between two slices of whole wheat bread.
- Add nuts or low-fat granola to your favorite yogurt.
- Try dried fruits for something new. These are higher in fiber than canned or whole fruits.
- Leave the skin or peel on fruits and vegetables when possible and wash them thoroughly before eating. Most of the fiber found in fruits and vegetables are in and around the skin.

- Read food labels and choose foods that are higher in fiber. Keep these nutritional claims in mind: "Good Source of Fiber" means three to less than five grams of fiber. "High in Fiber," "Rich in Fiber," and "Excellent Source of Fiber" mean five grams of fiber or more (20 percent or more of your daily value).

Your Nutrition Solution Tidbit

The market is loaded with fiber supplements. To get all of the benefits that fiber provides, don't take the easy way out. Whole foods provide more fiber as well as added essential nutrients such as vitamins, minerals, antioxidants, and phytonutrients that are necessary for optimal health. Never replace whole foods or any food group with a simple single supplement. Use fiber supplements as they are intended, to supplement your fiber intake and not to take the place of high fiber foods.

Say Good-Bye to Added Sugars

Added sugars are a big no-no when it comes to reducing inflammation. This includes anything from sugar-laden soft drinks and other beverages to your favorite candy bar or cookie and everything in between. The sugar that spikes in your blood from eating added sugars increases levels of the inflammatory markers called cytokines. Sugar can be found naturally in some foods including *lactose* in most dairy products and *fructose* in fruits. However, the majority of sugars found in the average American diet are added sugars. These sugars are added in processing, preparation, or at the table to sweeten and improve palatability. They are also added as a preservative and to provide texture, body, viscosity, and browning capacity to foods.

Although our body cannot determine the difference between natural and added sugars, the key is that foods with natural sugars usually contain the whole package of nutrients and other healthful components such as fiber, which can slow down the absorption of sugar into the blood stream. On the other hand, most foods with added sugars often supply calories with little to no essential nutrients and no fiber. You may see added sugars on food labels termed as high fructose corn syrup, white sugar, brown sugar, corn syrup, raw sugar, malt syrup, fructose sweetener, liquid fructose, honey, molasses, and crystal dextrose. The major sources of added sugars in the American diet include soft drinks, energy drinks, sports drinks, baked goods, sugar-sweetened drinks, dairy-based drinks, and candy. Reducing the consumption of added sugars can lower the calorie content of the diet without the worry of leaving out essential nutrients.

Added sugars are a particular concern in the American diet because they have been found to be consumed in excessive amounts and are associated with higher inflammation levels. In addition, added sugars can contribute a substantial amount of calories to our diets without contributing to our nutritional needs. This makes them very dangerous when it comes to managing weight as well as blood sugar. When consumed in excess, foods that contain added sugars begin to take the place of foods with essential vitamins, minerals, and fiber. Reducing the consumption of these foods allows us to increase our intake of nutrient-dense foods without going over our total daily calorie needs. Now let's be realistic: we can't stay away from our favorite sweets forever! But we can greatly reduce the intake of these added sugars and save these foods for an occasional treat instead of being part of our regular daily diet.

Step 3. Power Up on Plant Foods

The typical American diet is chock-full of animal foods and much too low in plant foods. Plant-based foods have loads of benefits including a lower risk for type 2 diabetes, heart disease, certain types of cancer, and hypertension, as well as better blood sugar control and weight management. Plant foods are loaded with vitamins, minerals, antioxidants, phytonutrients, fiber, and other healthy substances that are all associated with lower levels of pro-inflammatory markers.

Your Nutrition Solution Tidbit

Phytonutrients (or phytochemicals) are natural compounds found in plant foods including fruits, vegetables, grains, legumes, tree nuts, and teas that have strong antioxidant, immune-boosting, and other health-promoting properties. Some phytonutrients include carotenoids, flavonoids, isoflavones, lignans, indoles, and saponins, just to name a few.

Plant foods are the only foods where we get an abundance of anti-inflammatory phytonutrients. Now I am not saying that you must become a vegetarian, but you should consider taking a good look at your dietary intake and begin including more plant foods. Plant foods include whole grains of all kinds, legumes, dried beans, lentils, fruits, vegetables, nuts, seeds, and soy foods. There is hardly a lack of choice when it comes to these healthy, low-fat foods.

Your Nutrition Solution Tidbit

The American Cancer Institute for Cancer Research recommends filling at least 2/3 of your plate with plant foods. They recommend making 1/2 of your plate non-starch vegetables and fruits of all colors and varieties and 1/4 of your plate whole grains and starchy vegetables such as potatoes, corn, and peas.

The Soy Food Link

Soy foods and foods that contain soy protein can be found in just about every aisle of the supermarket these days. Soy foods originated from the simple soybean that itself can be consumed whole after being boiled or roasted. But because the protein in the soybean is so incredibly versatile, it has transformed into hundreds of different food products from hot dogs to yogurt to peanut butter. Soybeans are a power-house of nutritional value. They are rich in B-vitamins, iron, magnesium, potassium, and calcium as well as fiber in their whole form. The protein in these little powerhouses are the only plant food that is considered a "complete protein," which means they contain the correct ratio of essential amino acids for optimal use by our bodies, making them a high quality protein. Because most complete proteins are found only in animal foods, this makes soy a great source of protein without the cholesterol, saturated fats, and other corrupt components of animal foods. If that weren't enough, soybeans contain some essential fatty acids including omega-6 and omega-3. In fact, some soy foods such as edamame (whole green soy-beans) contain very high amounts of omega-3 fat in the form of alpha-linolenic acid (ALA), which has been found to reduce inflammation and reduce risk of heart disease.

With this superior nutritional profile, it isn't surprising that soy has some great health benefits including helping to lower LDL (bad cholesterol) and increase HDL (good cholesterol), lowering triglyceride levels, improving heart health, decreasing risk for certain types of cancer, relieving menopausal symptoms, and helping to prevent osteoporosis.

Experts believe that most of the beneficial effects of soy foods can be attributed to a compound called *phytoestrogens*, in particular *isoflavones*. The main isoflavones found in soy include *genistein* and *daidzien*. Although soy research still has much to uncover, the nutrient profile of soy proves that it deserves a role in the American diet that tends to be too high in saturated fat and cholesterol, mainly in the form of animal proteins.

What have the studies uncovered concerning soy and inflammation? A 2014 study in the *European Journal of Nutrition* concluded that anti-inflammatory properties of component(s) of soy protein may be a possible mechanism for the prevention of chronic inflammatory diseases such as atherosclerosis. Another study in 2012 in the *Journal of Academy of Nutrition and Dietetics* found that soy products had a marked anti-inflammatory effect. The possible mechanisms proposed for reducing inflammation are the phytoestrogens and/or the omega-3 fatty acids found in soy foods. The FDA has even approved a health claim on packaged food labels that states, "25 grams of soy protein a day, as part of a low in saturated fat and cholesterol, may reduce the risk of heart disease."

Your Nutrition Solution Tidbit

Due to some of the hormone-like compounds found in soy foods, if you have a hormone-sensitive condition, such as breast cancer or endometriosis, check with your doctor before including and/or increasing soy in your daily diet.

As healthy as soy foods can be, they are not without their controversies. Questions have been raised in concern about soy foods and their safety in relation to breast cancer, thyroid health, and other hormonal effects due to the phytoestrogens that soy foods contain. However, science is finding that soy foods in moderation are perfectly safe and can be beneficial to health. Your best bet, for maximum health benefits, is to choose primarily whole soy foods such as edamame, tofu, tempeh, soy milk, soy nuts, and "cheeses" that are made from soybeans. Some processed soy ingredients such as isolated soy protein that you find in many nutritional bars, snack foods, protein drinks, and soy isolate found in imitation meats leave out many of the nutritional components found in whole soy foods that incorporate soy's healthiest benefits.

Your Nutrition Solution Tidbit

Phytoestrogens are chemical compounds found naturally in soybeans (as genistein) that have estrogen-like properties.

Tips to Powering Up on Plant Foods

- At least once a week, substitute your meat dish for one made with plant foods such as soybeans, legumes/beans, and lentils.
- Include some type of fruit and vegetable, or both, at every meal.
- Choose oatmeal or a whole grain cereal for breakfast and add fruit, raisins, and ground flaxseed to it.
- Switch your fat-free milk for a light soy milk.
- Add legumes or dried beans to casseroles, salads, and soups.
- Use beans in place of ground beef in tacos, casserole, chili, or burritos.
- Use a nut butter, such as almond butter, on whole grain toast or bagel for breakfast or a great energy-boosting snack.
- Load your pizza with all veggies instead of any high fat meats.
- Use pureed avocado as a topping for sandwiches instead of mayo or as a topping for grilled chicken or as a dip for veggies.
- Look up some great recipes for green or fruit smoothies online and try incorporating them a few times a week for a meal or snack.
- Serve a salad as a meal several times throughout the week. Load on fresh veggies, dark greens, seeds, and a healthy dressing.
- Plan ahead and think of ways you can incorporate *more* plant foods into your diet every day in place of animal foods. It won't be as hard as you think!

Your Nutrition Solution Tidbit

Unfortunately, soy foods aren't right for everyone. Many people, especially people with irritable bowel syndrome (IBS), carry an intolerance or sensitivity to soy foods and can experience discomfort after eating them. If you suffer from IBS or find that soy foods are problematic for you, then it makes sense to limit them in your diet and find other ways to include plant foods.

Step 4. Shoot for a Healthy Weight

Obesity has now been added to the group of diseases that are known to present a low-grade inflammatory response such as type 2 diabetes, metabolic syndrome, and other chronic conditions. What is of even more concern is visceral fat or fat that accumulates around the abdominal area. This type of fat, in particular, is associated with low grade inflammation that contributes to metabolic disease, insulin resistance, and atherosclerosis or the build-up of plaque in the arteries. Researchers are learning that visceral fat produces pro-inflammatory cytokines that increase the risk of cardiovascular disease and other chronic health conditions. When high levels of body fat, especially visceral fat, are combined with physical inactivity, poor nutrition, and advancement in age, the health effects are even more prominent.

The good news is that making these lifestyle changes, including weight loss, can reverse this. Losing just 10 percent of your current body weight can reduce inflammation by reducing the pro-inflammatory chemicals in the blood. In turn, this positive change can begin to reverse health conditions from lowering blood pressure to lowering LDL cholesterol. If you are already at a healthy weight, then the goal is to maintain that weight. If you are overweight or obese, then the goal is to slowly and steadily lose weight in a healthy manner, no more than one to two pounds per week. Always check with your doctor first to discuss the weight-loss strategy that is best for you and to be thoroughly checked out before starting any type of weight loss plan.

Determine Your Healthy Weight

You realize that you need to lose weight, but exactly how much? How do I know what my healthy weight really should be? Body Mass Index (BMI) is one way to determine if your extra pounds translate into greater health risk. BMI is the measurement of your weight relative to your height and can determine whether you are at a healthy weight or if your weight is possibly contributing to poor health, including chronic inflammation. Keep in mind that BMI is not a measurement of body fat; therefore, it can sometimes misclassify people. For example, people with a lot of muscle mass may have a BMI that shows too high because BMI doesn't measure exact body fat and doesn't take into consideration that the majority of their body weight is coming from muscle and not fat. It can do the opposite for elderly people and underestimate BMI, not taking into account the muscle mass they have lost through the years. However, for the majority of us, BMI is a good general indicator of what our healthy weight range should be and if we are putting ourselves at risk for health issues related to our weight.

You can crunch the numbers yourself by using this formula:

Weight in pounds ÷ [height in inches]^2 x 703

You can also find calculators online such as *www.choosemyplate.gov/supertracker-tools/resources/bmi-calculator.html*.

Or you can use the following chart* to easily find your BMI:

BMI	19	20	21	22	23	24	25	26	27	28	29	30	31	32	33	34	35
Height									Weight in Pounds								
4'10"	91	96	100	105	110	115	119	124	129	134	138	143	148	153	158	162	167
4'11"	94	99	104	109	114	119	124	128	133	138	143	148	153	158	163	168	173
5'	97	102	107	112	118	123	128	133	138	143	148	153	158	163	168	174	179
5'1"	100	106	111	116	122	127	132	137	143	148	153	158	164	169	174	180	185
5'2"	104	109	115	120	126	131	136	142	147	153	158	164	169	175	180	186	191
5'3"	107	113	118	124	130	135	141	146	152	158	163	169	175	180	186	191	197
5'4"	110	116	122	128	134	140	145	151	157	163	169	174	180	186	192	197	204
5'5"	114	120	126	132	138	144	150	156	162	168	174	180	186	192	198	204	210
5'6"	118	124	130	136	142	148	155	161	167	173	179	186	192	198	204	210	216
5'7"	121	127	134	140	146	153	159	166	172	178	185	191	198	204	211	217	223
5'8"	125	131	138	144	151	158	164	171	177	184	190	197	203	210	216	223	230
5'9"	128	135	142	149	155	162	169	176	182	189	196	203	209	216	223	230	236
5'10"	132	139	146	153	160	167	174	181	188	195	202	209	216	222	229	236	243
5'11"	136	143	150	157	165	172	179	186	193	200	208	215	222	229	236	243	250
6'	140	147	154	162	169	177	184	191	199	206	213	221	228	235	242	250	258
6'1"	144	151	159	166	174	182	189	197	204	212	219	227	235	242	250	257	265
6'2"	148	155	163	171	179	186	194	202	210	218	225	233	241	249	256	264	272
6'3"	152	160	168	176	184	192	200	208	216	224	232	240	248	256	264	272	279
6'4"	156	164	172	180	189	197	205	213	221	230	238	246	254	263	271	279	287
	Healthy Weight						Overweight					Obese					

BMI	Weight
Below 18.5	Underweight
18.5 to 24.9	Healthy Weight
25.0 to 29.9	Overweight
Over 30.0	Obese

Source: Evidence Report of Clinical Guidelines on the Identification, Evaluation, and Treatment of Overweight and Obesity in Adults, 1998. NIH/National Heart, Lung, and Blood Institute (NHLBI) or check out: www.nhlbi.nih.gov/guidelines/obesity/bmi_tbl.htm for additional heights and weights.

To use this BMI chart, locate your height in the left-hand column and follow the row across that height to find your weight. Follow that column of the weight up to the top to locate your BMI. Now that you know your BMI, what exactly does it mean? Healthy weight is a range and not one single weight. The following will show you what range you fall into and what your BMI means for you.

Your Nutrition Solution Tidbit

BMI for children and adolescents is used slightly differently. Because they are continually growing, their BMI is instead plotted on a growth chart. The percentile indicates the relative position of a child's BMI compared to that among children of the same gender and age.

Does My Body Shape Matter?

BMI is only one factor in the attempt to assess your weight. For an accurate assessment of weight related to health, it is also important to look at where you store fat. In typical nutrition fashion, the shape of our bodies or where we store that excess fat, are compared to fruit, either an apple or a pear shape.

If you are shaped more like an apple, meaning you store and carry the majority of your fat in the stomach area and around your waist, you are at a higher risk for certain health problems such as cardiovascular disease, high blood pressure, type 2 diabetes, and certain types of cancer as well as chronic inflammation.

If you are shaped more like a pear, meaning you store and carry the majority of your fat below the waist, in your hips, buttocks, and thighs, your shape does not put you at as much of a health risk as storing fat in other regions. This doesn't mean you don't need to drop that extra weight, but the good news is it doesn't put you at as high a risk for health issues related to weight.

Most of us are painfully aware of where we store every little bit of fat, so you shouldn't have much of a problem figuring out what type of fruit you resemble. But if you just can't decide whether you look more like an apple or a pear, you can use your waist-to-hip ratio. Your waist-to-hip ratio can help determine, in a more scientific way, if the location of your body fat is putting you at greater risk for health problems related to your weight.

Follow these steps to figure out your waist-to-hip ratio:

1. Stand relaxed. Measure your waist at its smallest point (just above your hip bone) without sucking in your stomach or pulling the tape measure too tight.

2. Measure your hips by measuring the largest part of your buttocks and hips.

3. Divide your waist measurement by your hip measurement.

4. If this number is nearly or more then 1.0, you would be considered an apple shape.

5. If this number is considerably less than 1.0, you would be considered a pear shape.

Why is this important to you? The more body fat you carry in the stomach and waist area, the more at risk you are for chronic inflammation and all of the chronic health issues that are associated with it. The more weight you gain, the more health issues you will most likely encounter.

Your Nutrition Solution Tidbit

Your body shape, whether apple or pear, can be an inherited gene. In other words, where you carry body fat can be something that is passed down through your family tree and something you don't have a whole lot of control over. But you do have control over how much excess fat you have on your body to be stored. Your goal should be to reach a healthy weight to decrease the stored fat, whether you are an apple or a pear.

Steps to Taking It off for Good

There are so many necessary reasons to reach a healthy weight. If you are reading this book, reducing or preventing chronic inflammation is probably at the top of your list. If you are far from your healthy weight range, take heart in knowing that a little bit can go a long way. If you are on the overweight side of the coin, losing just 5 to 10 percent of your current weight can sometimes be just the ticket to improve your health and health-related conditions. But you can't stop there! Reaching your healthy weight once and for all will not only help to get your health under control, but it will most likely end up helping in ways you never even thought of.

If you are like most people, you want to lose weight the quickest and easiest way possible. Who doesn't? But resist the urge to sign up for fad diets or any type of diet that promises quick and easy weight loss. These types of diets usually revolve around deprivation of some type and can easily deplete your body's stores of essential nutrients; not to mention that losing weight too quickly is usually the weight loss that never sticks.

Steer clear of liquid diets, diet pills, or diet supplements that promise that tempting quick fix. Slow and steady wins the race to long-lasting weight loss, reduced inflammation, and overall better health. Losing one to two pounds per week is a safe and effective goal. The ultimate goal should be to lose the weight and keep it off for good!

It doesn't take as much change as you think to begin losing weight. You can do it safely by adding or subtracting as little as 250 to 500 calories per day. That can be as simple as eliminating a regular can of soda and that midday candy bar, and as we know, neither of these do inflammation any justice anyhow! There is no need to drastically slash your food intake all at one time or change your entire diet. Instead, make changes and cut back slowly. Making healthier choices by eliminating unhealthy foods and replacing them with healthier foods, as we discussed earlier in this chapter, will automatically cut calorie intake most of the time. As you lose weight and your body becomes accustomed to this new calorie level, which you might notice by experiencing a weight plateau, it may be time to make a few more changes and cut back a bit more. The idea is that for a permanent weight loss, you want to lose weight slowly, steadily, and in a healthy manner. Like we talked about before, it doesn't take much to begin reversing the process and getting yourself on track.

Your Nutrition Solution Tidbit

About 3,500 calories add up to one pound. Therefore, to lose one pound per week you need to split up a deficit of 3,500 calories over a week's time. Deducting 500 calories per day should result in a one pound per week weight loss.

The key is to worry less about every little calorie and con-centrate more in general on eating nutrient-rich foods that make calories count while still keeping an eye on your portion sizes, which will keep control of your calorie intake. This will ensure that even though you are trying to lose weight, you will still be getting all of the essential nutrients your body needs for good health. It is time to change bad habits into good ones and that goes for eating as well as exercise. Here are just a few strat-egies that may help you lose weight in a way that is healthy and lowers your risk for chronic inflammation:

- Your first order of business should be to truly consider your reasons for wanting to lose weight. Because you are reading this book, it is a good bet that reducing inflammation and all of the health is-sues and symptoms related to it, without the need for numerous and long-term medications, will be somewhere on that list. Knowing exactly what will motivate you and keep you committed to your goals *is* what will ultimately make you successful in your endeavor! To stay committed to your motiva-tions, write them down and look at them when you need that extra boost to keep you going.

- Secondly, you need to set goals. Set both short-term and long-term goals. Short-term goals are essen-tial to keep you going on the journey to reach your long-term goal of a healthy weight. Your goals need to be realistic, specific, and measurable. Write them down, along with your motivations, so you always know what you are working toward. Don't expect to change *all* of your bad habits, or the habits that have caused that extra weight gain, all at one time. Work on changing a few habits at a time. Once you have mastered one goal, move on to the next.

- Keep a daily food diary that includes what you eat, when you eat, and how much you eat. Write it down or find a free online food diary such as the Food Tracker on ChooseMyPlate.gov or a good app on your phone. Review your food diary frequently so that you can pinpoint and work on problem areas. Keeping a food diary will help to keep you compliant and on track.

- Get in the habit of being aware of every food and beverage you put in your mouth. Make yourself accountable for what you eat and the way you live your life. Concentrate on eating for true hunger and for properly fueling your body.

- Do *not* skip meals and that includes breakfast. You won't save calories. Skipping a meal will lead to eating more than you should at the next meal and/or cause uncontrolled snacking throughout the day, both of which will pack on more calories than you need, not to mention cause blood sugar levels to surge. Eating breakfast, especially if it is a whole grain cereal, is associated with better weight loss and blood sugar control.

- Stick to a well-balanced and healthy eating routine. Healthier choices usually mean fewer calories, less fat, less sodium, and more nutritional value. Become familiar with the Mediterranean diet and the USDA's Dietary Guidelines for Americans, both of which can help you to lose weight safely and reduce chronic inflammation.

- Cut out junk foods such as candy, cookies, cake, pies, other sweets, soft drinks, fast foods, and chips. Eating them occasionally is okay, but frequently causes weight gain and can trigger inflammation.

- Plan your healthy meals and snacks ahead of time so that you are always prepared.

- Include lots of fiber in your daily diet. We already know fiber may help you to reduce inflammation plus better manage blood sugar levels, but it can also be helpful with weight loss. High fiber meals and snacks help fill you up and keep you feeling fuller longer. Check back to earlier in the chapter on how to incorporate more fiber into your diet.

- Practice and become aware of portion control. Keep your portions more moderate and don't over-fill your stomach. Eat until you are comfortable, not stuffed.

- Avoid eating in front of the television, computer, or while doing other activities that keep you from paying attention to how much you are eating.

- Get in the habit of slowing yourself down while eating. It takes a good 20 minutes for your brain to get the message that you are full. Eating too quickly leads to overeating, which can lead to excess weight. Eating slower can result in eating less.

- Use a smaller size plate to dish up your food. It will help to keep your portions and calories under control and make you feel that you are getting a full plate of food. Just don't go back for seconds!

- Plan and prepare more meals at home to keep from eating out too often. Restaurant meals tend to be higher in calories, fat, and sodium and it can sometimes be too tempting to make the right choices when eating out. Don't deprive yourself of eating out, but make it an occasional outing instead of a regular habit, and work on making better choices when you do eat out.

- Learn how to read and use the Nutrition Facts Panel on food labels to your advantage. The Nutrition Facts Panel will help you to choose foods that best fit into your goals. It will provide you with a good measurement of portion sizes and calorie intake. We will discuss more about food labels in Chapter 5.

- Check out the USDA's ChooseMyPlate.gov Website to explore all of the information and hands-on tools that can help you lose weight sensibly and at the same time teach you what good nutrition really means.

- Incorporate some type of physical activity most days of the week. Overweight and obesity are direct results of an imbalance between the calories you take in and the calories you burn. It's just that simple. The more active you are, the more calories you will burn. Something as simple as walking can be a great start.

- Drink plenty of water throughout each day. Staying properly hydrated is essential to digestion and the fat burning process.

- If you feel you need more personal guidance, and many people do, turn to a Registered Dietitian (RD) or Registered Dietitian Nutritionist (RDN) who can educate, guide, motivate, and keep you on track to future success. You can check out *www.eatright.org* to find a dietitian in your area.

These simple tips and changes can help you improve your health, lose weight, and reduce inflammation. It is all about lifestyle change and making permanent changes that you can and will stick with for life. Once you begin to lose weight and feel better, you will be motivated to push ahead and finish your journey.

Step 5. Get Active

Exercise is a lifestyle habit that plays an extremely important role in managing and reaching a healthy weight and overall better health. Exercise doesn't need to mean hours at the gym, it can mean anything that helps to get your body moving. The goal is to get active and stay active on a regular basis with a solid exercise plan that both fits you and your lifestyle. Exercise boasts an endless list of health benefits, including improved insulin resistance, better blood sugar control, improved heart health, lowered LDL and increased HDL, improved sleep quality, better immune function, lowered blood pressure; protection against metabolic syndrome, weight loss and weight maintenance, decreased stress, and the list goes on.

But one very important benefit is that there is mounting evidence that regular exercise helps to reduce and possibly eliminate inflammation. Exercising at about 60 to 80 percent of your maximum heart rate, which for example would be briskly walking where you can still talk but can't quite carry on a conversation, can help to lower CRP (C-reactive protein), one of the key pro-inflammation markers. It also induces an increase in cytokines, an anti-inflammatory marker. Exercise is one lifestyle change that hands down correlates with better health in all studies. The key is to start moving and stay moving!

Your Nutrition Solution Tidbit

According to the Dietary Guidelines for Americans, adults aged 18 to 64 years should do at least two hours and 30 minutes (or 150 minutes) each week of aerobic activity at a moderate level *or* one hour and 15 minutes (or 75 minutes) each week of aerobic physical activity at a vigorous level. Being active five or more hours weekly can provide even more health benefits. Spreading your exercise over at least three days is suggested. Each activity should be done for at least 10 minutes at a time. Adults should also engage in resistance/strength training activities such as push-ups, sit-ups, and/or lifting weights at least two days per week.

Get Motivated and Stick With It

With all of the benefits right in front of you, it is pretty hard to say "no" to exercise! For some it will still take a bit of motivation to get started and especially to stick with it. Here are a few tips to help you do just that:

- Don't start with going all out. That can set you up for failure. Instead, set small, specific, and attainable goals for yourself, and once you reach a goal, set a new one. The idea is to keep moving ahead and to take small steps.

- Keep yourself motivated by the way you feel! Losing weight and just feeling physically better can sometimes be all the motivation you need. Take physical note of weight loss and other positives you notice, such as feeling better overall (both mentally and physically), feeling less fatigued, having less pain in joint areas, and sleeping better through the night.

- Do something you enjoy so that you are more apt to stick with it. Exercise doesn't mean hours at the gym; it means getting your body moving at a good pace on a regular basis. You can try swimming, dancing, tennis, running/jogging, walking, yoga, spinning, biking, hiking, or whatever else you enjoy doing!

- Schedule your daily exercise on your weekly calendar like you would do for all other weekly activities. Mark it on a calendar that you check daily.
- Use visual cues to both remind and motivate yourself. Stick a note on the refrigerator or your computer, or put your workout shoes by the door that you always use.
- Get a workout buddy and do it together.

Your Nutrition Solution Tidbit

Don't overdo a good thing! Going way over your current intensity level or basically over-exercising can lead to a pro-inflammatory response from your body—another good reason to start slowly and work your way up. Moderate exercise is key.

Guidelines for Getting Started

Before you get started, whether you have never exercised or are an avid exerciser, it is always a good idea to speak with your doctor first about what is safe for you and your individual situation. It is important to have a few guidelines and warnings under your belt before you do get started.

- Aim for 30 minutes of moderate-to-vigorous intensity aerobic activity at least five days per week for a total of 150 minutes per week.
- Aim for strength training at least two times per week, in addition to your aerobic exercise.
- If you have never exercised before, start slow and work your way up. Start with five to 10 minutes a

day and work up from there. Over time, your fitness will improve, and you will be able to do more for a longer period of time.

- For consistency, spread your physical activity out during the week so that you are able to exercise most days. Try to not go more than two days in a row without exercising.

- If you can't find the time for a block of 30 minutes, then split it up into three 10-minute increments throughout your day.

- Don't just rely on exercise for physical activity. Work more activity into your everyday life. Use the stairs, clean the house, walk the dog, wash the car—they all add up.

- The best time to eat is about 30 minutes before you exercise. You don't need an entire meal; a snack made up of at least 30 grams of carb and some protein will do, such as half a whole grain bagel with peanut butter or a banana and a handful of nuts. This will help you to better fuel your workout.

- Drink plenty of water before, during, and after exercise.

Your Nutrition Solution Tidbit

If you suffer from an inflammatory condition that involves joint pain, be sure to check with your doctor before starting an exercise program. You may need to consult with a personal trainer or physical therapist to tailor your workouts until you get to a point of less pain. Swimming can be a great exercise for those with joint issues.

Make Exercise Count

It is vital to an effective anti-inflammatory workout program to make certain you are working hard enough but not too hard. Another word for this is intensity or how hard your body is working during aerobic activity. You can test yourself in a few ways. One quick way is the "talk test." If you can comfortably carry on a conversation while exercising, you are working out at a moderate intensity and reaping the health benefits of the activity. The next step is a vigorous activity level where your heart rate goes up even more and you are breathing hard and fast, making it hard to hold a conversation. A mix of the two is a good combination, once you get to that level. Start at a lower intensity level and work your way up to a more vigorous one through time. If you get to the point that you can barely catch your breath and cannot carry on a conversation, you need to slow yourself down. On the other hand, if you can babble along without barely taking a breath in between sentences, then you need to step it up. You should feel like you are working yourself, but not to the point of pure exhaustion.

There is a more technical way to measure whether you are working out hard enough or too hard. Using a mathematical equation, you can calculate your target heart rate or the number of times your heart beats per minute. This will inform you whether you are working out at your target heart rate zone. According to the American Heart Association, the general target zone rate falls between 50 and 85 percent of your maximum heart rate. This is only an estimate, but will let you know whether you are working out too hard or not hard enough.

To calculate target heart rate zone:

1. Calculate your estimated maximum heart rate: 220 minus your age.

2. Calculate your lower range: Maximum heart rate multiplied by .50 (50 percent).

3. Calculate your upper range: Maximum heart rate multiplied by .85 (85 percent).

EXAMPLE: 30-Year-Old Woman

1. 220 − 30 = 190 maximum heart rate

2. 190 × .50 = 95 lower range

3. 190 × .85 = 162 upper range

This means that her target zone is between 95 and 162 beats per minute. So if she falls below 95, then she needs to step it up, and if she goes higher than 162, she needs to ease up. If you are a beginning exerciser or have not exercised in quite some time, aim for the lower range of your target rate. As you become more physically fit, you will be able to gradually build up to the higher end.

To keep yourself in your target zone, you need to check your heart rate throughout your exercise session. To find your pulse, place your index and middle fingers over the outside of your opposite wrist and press lightly. Once you have located your pulse, use the second hand of a watch or clock and count the beats you feel in a 15-second span. Multiply that number by four. That is your heart rate at that moment in time.

Types of Exercise Activities

There is never a shortage of fun and beneficial ways to exercise. The key is to choose something that suits you and that you enjoy doing. This will help you to stay motivated and stick with it. No matter what you choose, always warm up for at least five minutes before starting your exercise and cool down for five minutes afterward. The best type of exercise program combines both aerobic and strength training.

Aerobic Activity

The word aerobic literally means "with air." Therefore, in aerobic exercise your muscles require an increased supply of oxygen. Aerobic activity is also known as cardio activity because it also speeds your heart rate and improves your lung and heart fitness. Aerobic exercise helps your body to better utilize insulin. It strengthens your heart, relieves stress, improves circulation, lowers blood pressure, and reduces inflammation, just to name a few. Doing a combination of different aerobic exercise during your week helps to keep exercise more interesting and move all the different parts of your body.

Examples of aerobic exercise include:

- Brisk walking.
- Swimming or water aerobics.
- Dancing.
- Biking/spinning.
- Jogging/running.
- Stair climbing.
- Low-impact aerobics.
- Rowing.
- Cross-country skiing.
- Tennis.
- Cardio machines, such as a cross trainer or elliptical machine.

Strength or Resistance Training

This type of activity helps to build and maintain muscles and bones by working them against gravity. Strength training is used for improving muscle strength and tone. In men, it will increase muscle size; for women, it usually means more tone without significant muscle size increase. Strength training or resistance training makes your body more sensitive to insulin and can help to lower blood glucose as well as maintain and build muscle and strengthen bones. The more muscle you have, the higher your metabolism or the more calories you burn all the time, not just when exercising. Strength training can include using free weights such as dumbbells and weight machines or stretch bands for resistance training. It can also include exercises that use your own body weight—such as lunges, squats, and push-ups—or classes that involve strength training.

Stretching and Flexibility

Stretching, flexibility, and balance exercises are another form of exercise to include in your routine. This type of activity can include something as easy as basic stretches to yoga, Pilates, and tai chi. Stretching and flexibility can help to stretch out joints and prevent stiffness, especially for those suffering with any form of arthritis. Gentle stretching for five to 10 minutes before and after exercise is great for warm up and cool down, and helps prevent injury. These can all be great for stress relief as well. Balance or stability exercises are beneficial for any age, but especially for those that are aging and starting to lose some balance. These types of exercises can help you stay steady on your feet and reduce the risk of falling and being injured. Examples include walking backward or sideways, standing on one leg at a time, and standing from a sitting position. Exercises that strengthen your leg muscles and your lower core muscles are also good for balance. If your balance isn't great, make sure to have someone spot you as you do these exercises.

No matter what you decide to include in your exercise program, a well-balanced exercise routine should include a combination of aerobic exercise, resistance or strength training, and flexibility/stretching/balance.

Daily Lifestyle Activity Counts

Exercise is not the only way to burn calories and keep your body, muscles, and joints moving. In addition to exercise, think about how else you can keep yourself moving throughout the day. In the electronic and convenient world we live in today, it isn't always easy to get more activity in through lifestyle. But if you make an effort, you can keep yourself moving all day long!

Here are a few ideas to get you started and keep you going:

- Take the stairs instead of the elevator.
- Park at the far end of the parking lot for a longer walk, but be safe.
- Forget the drive-thru at the bank or the pharmacy; park and walk in.
- If you have a sit-down job, get up every 30 minutes or less and move around.
- Play actively with your kids instead of watching from the sidelines.
- Take the dog for regular walks.
- Wash the car yourself instead of taking it to the car wash.
- While on the phone, walk around the house instead of sitting on the couch.
- Mow the grass, rake the leaves, and work out in the garden.

Your Nutrition Solution Tidbit

Using a pedometer to monitor how many steps you take a day can be a great way to get started with physical activity or as an addition to your exercise plan. An article in the *Harvard Health Letter* states that a summary of 26 different studies found that people who use pedometers actually increase their activity by almost 30 percent. Having a goal of 10,000 steps a day (about five miles) is important. You don't have to reach that goal at the beginning, but work your way up to it.

More Helpful Lifestyle Changes

We have discussed some very doable diet and lifestyle changes that you can start right now and that will make a world of difference in eliminating, preventing, and reducing chronic inflammation. But why stop there? There are even more changes that will make a difference in your current and future health status.

Stop Smoking

The World Health Organization (WHO) states that cigarette smoking is one of the single largest preventable causes of disease and premature death. Smoking is a major contributor to heart disease, stroke, hypertension, chronic lung disease, cancer, and so much more. Smoking cigarettes triggers a response that increases levels of pro-inflammatory markers, including CRP. Stopping the smoking habit can be a tremendous benefit to chronic pain due to inflammatory conditions, and can prevent and reduce chronic inflammation in general, as well as prevent further health damage. If you are determined to get healthier and leave inflammation and all its health issues and pain behind, then quitting smoking needs to be at the top of the list.

Here are some tips to help you quit:

- Choose a day you are going to quit and stick with it. Do not choose a day that is too soon or too far away. Use that short time before to get prepared and have an action plan.

- Find your support system. This can be family, friends, or others that are trying to quit. Let them know the day you have decided to quit and ask for their support. Let those people know how they can best help you.

- Prepare yourself for quitting day by going through your house, car, purse, etc. and getting rid of all tobacco products, ashtrays, lighters, or any other object tied to your smoking.

- Have an action plan by going through your day and noting the day-to-day activities that trigger your urge for a cigarette. Make plans to deal with those times in a different way.

- Focus on getting healthier by eating healthy and getting active.

- Speak with your doctor about your plans and ask about possible nicotine-replacing products that can help you get through the rough patches.

- Join a support group where there are other people trying to kick the habit. A support group can help get you through the rough times and offer some much needed assistance and advice.

Your Nutrition Solution Tidbit

According the U.S. Centers for Disease Control (CDC), tobacco smoke contains a deadly mix of more than 7,000 chemicals, with hundreds of them being toxic. At least 70 of those chemicals are known to cause cancer, not just in the lungs, but anywhere in the body. For more information, visit *http://smokefree.gov/*.

Get More Sleep

Believe it or not, poor sleep habits can be a cause for inflammation. Pro-inflammatory cytokines are produced at a higher rate by those people who do not get enough sleep every night on a regular basis. While we sleep, our body regenerates and the immune system calms down. Lack of sleep, and therefore of this restorative process, is a major promoter of chronic inflammation. Many people with rheumatoid arthritis, fibromyalgia, or other autoimmune disorders are in a vicious cycle; they lose sleep due to pain associated with their condition, which tends to promote flare-ups and more pain.

The goal should be to clock in at least six to eight hours of restful sleep each night. A study by a group of U.S. researchers presented by Dr. Alanna Morris, a cardiology fellow at Emory University School of Medicine in Atlanta at the American Heart Association 2010 Scientific Sessions found undoubtedly that poor sleep quality and not getting enough sleep are both linked to higher levels of chronic inflammation. Three pro-inflammatory markers were evaluated in studies and all three, including CRP, IL-6, and fibrinogen, were significantly higher in people who had less than six hours of sleep and had poor sleep quality. In fact, they concluded that poor sleep quality and short sleep durations could increase the risk of heart disease and stroke through chronic inflammation. If sleep time is a problem for you on a regular basis, it is time to get some help and improve your health.

Here are a few tips to get you started:

- First of all, visit your doctor. Be sure there is not a medical or medication reason why you are unable to get a full night's sleep. Your doctor might recommend a sleep study to evaluate your sleeping habits.

- Do your best to stick to a regular bedtime.

- Turn off the computer, phones, tablets, television, or any other electronic device you have at least an hour before bedtime. Watching these right before bedtime can increase brain activity and make sleep difficult.

- Do something relaxing before you go to sleep such as yoga, meditation, reading (a paper book and not on a screen), soothing music, etc.

- Try not to nap during the day so you will be more tired at night.

- Do not drink alcohol or caffeine containing products too close to bedtime.

- If you can't turn off your thoughts, write them down each night before bedtime as a way to get them off your mind until the next day.

- Do not take sleeping medication unless you speak with your doctor first. Many can be addictive and create a whole new problem for you.

Getting enough sleep will not only help you to combat inflammation, but it will boost the immune system, increase energy levels, help to decrease chronic pain, put you in a better mood, lead to clearer thinking, and possibly lead to better weight control. For more information, visit *http://sleepfoundation.org/*.

Keep Stress to a Minimum

Being stressed-out frequently will not only lead to gray hair, but may also open the door to chronic inflammation. Chronic stress can wreak havoc on not just our emotions and our mind, but on our physical body as well. It can lead to issues such as depression, headaches, weight gain, stomach issues, anxiety, panic attacks, stiff neck and shoulders, and an increased heart rate. Through time, stress can lead to a compromised immune system, heart disease, acid reflux, serious stomach issues, infertility, skin problems, and more.

A research team led by Sheldon Cohen from Carnegie Mellon University found that psychological stress is directly associated with the body losing the ability to regulate the inflammatory response process, creating increased levels of inflammation in the body. We all get stressed out from time to time, but it may be time to evaluate your stress levels. If you feel chronic stress is an issue for you, it's time to learn some coping strategies that will help decrease your stress levels before they hurt you physically.

Here are a few tips to help you out:

- Start a regular exercise program. This is a great stress reliever and, as an added bonus, can help you shed pounds and prevent or reduce chronic inflammation.
- Write down your feelings and thoughts in a journal. Sometimes getting thoughts down on paper can get them off your mind and help you relax.

- Look at your daily schedule and see how you can slow down a bit by letting people help you with daily tasks.
- Meditate daily in a quiet area. Focus on the present and on your breathing. It can be tough at first, but you will eventually learn to shut everything out during that time and relax deeply.
- Try a more meditational and relaxing type of yoga. Taking a class can help.
- Get a regular massage.
- Get adventurous and try alternative therapies, such as acupuncture or Reiki therapy.
- Adopt a new, relaxing hobby, such as gardening, reading, working with animals, or whatever says "relax" to you.
- If you don't feel you are able to de-stress, speak with your doctor about a possible referral to a counselor that can help you out on a one-to-one basis.

Your Nutrition Solution Tidbit

A 2010 study in the *Journal of Psychosomatic Medicine* found that women who practiced 75 to 90 minutes of Hatha Yoga twice weekly for at least two years were found to have significantly lower levels of IL-6 and CRP, two key inflammatory markers, compared to women who were just starting yoga or practiced less frequently.

chapter 4

10 foods to avoid and 10 foods to include for reducing inflammation

Food is a large part of reducing and eliminating chronic inflammation. Experts believe that anti-inflammatory benefits come from the synergistic effect of foods that are consumed together as well as from individual foods. They don't feel there is one specific anti-inflammatory "diet," but rather there are diets designed around the individual foods that are believed to reduce inflammation and the ones that are believed to increase inflammation. Just a few small changes of adding some of the right foods and avoiding some of the wrong foods can play a major role in managing inflammation. There are many food and beverage choices that are not considered the best because they may wreak havoc on inflammation. Some of them aren't necessarily "bad" foods or unhealthy (though some are), but they are just not the best choice for reducing inflammation. On the other hand, there are some really good choices that may do the opposite and help you manage chronic inflammation, as well as the pain and other symptoms and serious health conditions that accompany it. We will discuss some of these foods in this chapter to give you an idea of foods to include and those to avoid.

10 Common Culprits

We have discussed many components of different foods that are known to trigger inflammation including saturated fat, trans fat, added sugar, omega-6 fatty acids, refined carbo-hydrates, and dietary cholesterol. When you already have an inflammatory condition such as arthritis, eating foods that can trigger inflammation can make symptoms even worse. Even if you don't suffer from an inflammatory condition, eating foods that are inflammatory on a regular basis can cause health conditions down the road. The following are some individual foods or ingredients that can be major inflammatory triggers and ones you should avoid whether you already have known inflammation or not.

1. **Fast food.** Fast food can be detrimental to anyone's diet but can especially increase pro-inflammatory markers. Not only do most fast food meals contain loads of calories that can lead to weight gain, they are also loaded with sodium, cholesterol, trans fat, saturated fat, and refined carbs, and void of fiber and essential nutrients. Fried foods soak up tons of oil, leading to even more additional calories. However, all of us are busy people and on occasion eating on the run is a convenient option. If you find yourself in this situation, the key is to make healthier choices and not be tempted by the foods you know you should avoid. Stay away from "super-sizing" and look at nutritional information, which all fast food places now have, before you order. Avoid the foods and ingredients that you have learned can trigger chronic inflammation and stick with healthier options such as salads, grilled chicken, etc. Your best option, if you know you are going to be out and about, is to carry food with you or choose a fast food restaurant where you're sure you can get something healthier. Fast food

on occasion is one thing, but making a regular habit out of it can definitely lead to a host of health issues, including chronic inflammation.

2. **Alcohol.** Regular over-consumption of alcohol can have many negative health effects, from liver damage to heart disease to insulin resistance, all of which can increase or create inflammation. Prolonged and heavy use of alcohol can wreak havoc all over your body by increasing the production of cytokines and other pro-inflammatory markers. Because heavy drinkers usually have higher levels of the stress-response hormone cortisol in their body, they are more susceptible to depression, other addictions, and frequent mood changes. On the other hand, moderate consumption of alcoholic beverages, one drink per day for women and two drinks per day for men, seem to have an impact on lowering CRP, a powerful signal for inflammation. Keep in mind that red wine is a good choice because it contains a heart healthy and anti-inflammatory component called resveratrol. The key with alcohol is moderation. Drinking too much too often will most definitely cause health issues of all kinds and will promote chronic inflammation. If you feel you are drinking too much, see your doctor to discuss ways you can take back control. If you don't drink, then don't start because of probable health benefits.

Your Nutrition Solution Tidbit

One drink is equal to one 12-ounce beer, 8-ounce malt liquor, 5-ounce glass of wine, or 1.5 ounces of 80-proof distilled spirits or liquor.

---

3. **MSG.** MSG, or mono-sodium glutamate, is a processed flavor-enhancing additive that can be found in numerous popular processed foods such as canned soups, salad dressing, hot dogs, processed and packaged deli meats, frozen meals, canned spaghettis, gravy mixes, seasoning blends, snack foods, fast foods, Asian foods, and soy sauce, as well as many others. MSG can trigger multiple pathways of chronic inflammation, especially in the liver. In addition, MSG has a reputation for not only promoting inflammation but for triggering headaches (especially migraines for some people), as well as skin rashes, asthma, heart irregularities, and numerous others. The best way to combat MSG is to avoid it by buying whole, fresh foods and cooking at home as much as possible. Reading ingredient lists on packaged foods is helpful, but it is important to know you won't always see "MSG" on the label, even if the food contains it. Some of its alias names include autolyzed yeast, yeast extract, maltodextrin, hydrolyzed protein, sodium caseinate, mono-potassium glutamate, and textured protein.

4. **Deli meats.** We already know that many packaged deli meats contain MSG, an inflammatory promoter. In addition, some of these types of deli meats, especially ham, salami, and bologna, as well as bacon, jerky, and sausage, are commonly preserved with sodium nitrates, which help to prevent the growth of certain bacteria. Nitrates actually occur naturally in the environment (such as in soil or fresh water systems) and in some foods (such as root vegetables, spinach, and celery) and in the body they are converted to nitrites. In large amounts, these chemicals are known as a possible cancer-causing agent. In addition, nitrites can increase inflammation and contribute to the chronic disease

process. You can find nitrate-free deli meats if you do a little snooping and read the label on the back of meat packages. If the meat is in the deli and not labeled, never be afraid to ask questions. Because deli meats can be high in sodium and many times in saturated fats as well, your best bet is to stick with lean fresh meats or even tuna packed in water for sandwiches. This doesn't necessarily mean you should never eat deli meats again, but you should be mindful of the amount and frequency in which you eat them and take a better look at what is in the deli meats you purchase.

5. **Soft drinks.** Soft drinks (or "soda" and "pop" depending on where you live), whether diet or full of regular sugar, seem to be the drink of choice for many Americans these days. Soft drinks are what we dietitians call "empty calories," meaning these beverages provide calories but have absolutely no nutritional value. Besides the health effects that drinking too many soft drinks can lead to, going overboard can also be an easy way to put on the pounds, which as we know can lead to triggering chronic inflammation. These types of carbonated beverages do contain lots of other substances, none of them being good. They contain phosphoric acid, which has been shown to deplete calcium stores from our bones, leading to osteoporosis, weakened bones, and decreased bone mass. The average 12 ounce can of cola contains a whopping nine teaspoons of refined sugar, in the form of high fructose corn syrup, causing spikes in both blood sugar and insulin, which in turn can trigger chronic inflammation. Soft drinks are also associated with additional pain in already arthritic joints. And let's not forget the caffeine, especially in energy drinks, that can just compound the whole problem even further.

If you think switching to "diet" soft drinks will help you out, think again. Just because they take the sugar out doesn't mean they make a healthier beverage. Many artificial sweeteners, such as aspartame, act as a foreign substance to the body, causing it to react by attacking the chemical, which in turn can trigger an inflammatory response, especially if you are sensitive to any of these specific chemicals. Many beverages can fall under this category in addition to soft drinks, including the increasingly popular energy drinks, vitamin waters, flavored waters, sports drinks, juice drinks, sweetened ice tea, etc. Your best bet is to either avoid these altogether or, at least, drink them only on occasion. Stick with water, fat-free dairy or soy beverages, 100-percent juices, unsweetened hot or iced tea, and unsweetened coffee.

6. **Added salt.** We often use the words "salt" and "sodium" interchangeably, but they are really different terms with different meanings. Salt is the actual table salt we use to add to foods and sodium is an ingredient in table salt, along with chloride and iodine. Sodium is an important mineral that we need in our body for some very vital functions. The problem is when we consume too much sodium, which can cause high blood pressure for those that are sodium-sensitive and can exacerbate inflammatory conditions such as arthritis. Many foods in our diets already contain natural levels of sodium, such as vegetables, dairy products, and meats. The last thing we need is to add table salt to our foods or in cooking and/or to choose processed foods that are high in sodium. In addition, we get loads of sodium from restaurant foods, packaged foods, processed meats, canned foods, and from ingredients such as soy sauce, MSG, garlic salt, baking soda, and the list goes on. Check food labels for sodium content and keep in mind that federal

guidelines recommend consuming less than 2,300 mg of sodium daily (the amount in one teaspoon of table salt). Choosing fresh foods more often, choosing lower sodium foods from the grocery store, and refraining from using additional salt in cooking and at the table can all add up to a lower sodium intake and a reduced incidence of inflammation and other health issues.

Your Nutrition Solution Tidbit

Children two years old and older, and adults younger than 50 years of age should get less than 2,300 mg of sodium daily. People over age 50, African Americans, and those who have high blood pressure, diabetes, and chronic kidney disease should get less than 1,500 mg of sodium daily.

---

7. **Nightshades.** Nightshades can be questionable when it comes to inflammation, but are also worth mentioning. To begin, nightshades are a group of fruits and vegetables that have a higher alkaloid content. There are more than 2,800 species of these plants that grow in the shade of night. For years, experts have believed that nightshades aggravate some inflammatory conditions such as arthritis and possibly fibromyalgia. At this point, research has failed to show a definite scientific link between nightshades and symptoms. However, experts still believe that some people do have a certain sensitivity to alkaloids and that it just isn't common enough for there to be significant results in studies. It does seem that there are people who do have problems with nightshades while others don't, just like any other sensitivity to a food or food chemical.

The only way for you to know for sure if you have a problem with nightshades is to experiment with an elimination diet. That means taking the specific foods completely out of your diet to see if any of your symptoms improve. It is important to keep a detailed food and symptom diary and to consult with a registered dietitian nutritionist if you have questions or are having difficulties. You can also consider MRT testing that we discussed in Chapter 1. If you suffer with an autoimmune disease, arthritis, gout, osteoporosis, fibromyalgia, ongoing inflammation, or other inflammatory conditions, it may be worth trying an elimination diet to see if nightshades cause a problem for you.

The following are some of the most common fruits and vegetables that are part of the nightshade family:

- White potatoes (not sweet potatoes).
- Tomatoes.
- Eggplant.
- Sweet and hot peppers.
- Cayenne peppers.
- Paprika.
- Ground cherries.
- Goji berries.

8. **High Fructose Corn Syrup.** Although all sugars will spike blood sugar, high fructose corn syrup (HFCS) is one to watch because it is included in so many foods and has some very negative health implications. HFCS has been linked to higher calorie intake, weight gain, and the increase of insulin resistance and triglycerides. HFCS is comprised of 55 percent fructose and 45 percent glucose. Fructose is a natural sugar found in

fruits, which doesn't sound so bad and, when it is in fruit, isn't! But the problem in HFCS is that fructose, when unaccompanied by the natural fiber in fruit, is far more harmful to our health than even table sugar. High doses of this free fructose, found in HFCS, literally damages the intestinal lining enough for toxic gut bacteria and partially digested food proteins to enter our blood stream and trigger chronic inflammation. HFCS represents more than 40 percent of the caloric sweeteners that are added to foods and beverages and is the only caloric sweetener added to soft drinks in the United States.

There is no way of knowing how much HFCS is in a food or beverage, but you can read the ingredient list on the food label to give you a clue. If HFCS is one of the first ingredients listed, it is safe to assume that the product contains quite a bit. Your best option is to check labels and avoid foods and beverages that contain any amount of HFCS. Avoiding highly processed foods and sticking more with fresh whole foods can help you to avoid HFCS. Common foods that contain HFCS include regular soft drinks, syrups, breakfast cereals, fruit juices, popsicles, fruit-flavored yogurts, ketchup or BBQ sauces, canned and jarred pasta sauces, canned soup, and canned fruits (if in syrup), just to name a few.

9. **Candy and other sweet treats.** We all experience that sweet tooth from time to time, but if you are trying to reduce or eliminate chronic inflammation, it is best to refrain from turning to candy and other sweet treats that contain refined sugars to quench that need. High-sugary foods such as candy, cookies, donuts, cake, syrup, and soft drinks are again known as "empty calories" providing plenty of calories but little to no

nutritional value. Too many of these foods can play havoc on your blood sugar levels, your weight loss efforts, and can trigger the release of the pro-inflammatory messengers known as cytokines. Learn to satisfy your sweet tooth in other ways with high-quality carbs that contain nutrients and fiber such as fresh fruit, low-fat fruited yogurt, or fat-free chocolate milk. When eating a piece of fruit, pair it with a protein choice such as peanut butter, low-fat cheese, or nuts to reduce the impact to your blood sugar and to better satisfy your hunger.

10. **Red meats.** Who doesn't love a juicy burger or a sizzling steak? The problem, according to many experts, including a 2014 study inthe *American Journal of Clinical Nutrition,* is that greater red meat intake is associated with unfavorable plasma concentrations of inflammatory biomarkers. Substituting red meat with other sources of healthier protein foods is associated with a lower biomarker profile of inflammation. The solution is to decrease your intake of red meats as much as possible. When it comes to meat, stick more with chicken, poultry, fish/seafood, and lean cuts of pork, and eat red meat only on occasion as is promoted in the Mediterranean diet. Try other sources of protein including soy foods, legumes/beans, lentils, egg whites, and peanut butter. There's nothing wrong with making that juicy burger out of ground turkey breast or substituting that sizzling steak with a chunk of marinated pork tenderloin on the grill.

Your Nutrition Solution Tidbit

Even though foods and food derivatives such as wheat, gluten, corn, soy, and dairy products are not unhealthy foods and not generally inflammatory, they are foods that tend to be at the top of the offender list for food sensitivities, which in turn can trigger inflammation. Just about any food can be pro-inflammatory for an individual if they have a sensitivity or are reactive to a particular food or food ingredient.

10 Potential Helpers

Just as there are foods that are known culprits for inflammation, there are also foods, beverages, herbs, and spices that can be helpful in keeping inflammation at bay. That doesn't mean that one specific food will do the magic trick for you, but adding these foods to an already healthy anti-inflammatory meal plan can make an even bigger impact. Keep in mind, though, that just because a food is generally anti-inflammatory in nature, doesn't mean it will be that way for everyone. Some people are sensitive to certain foods that can make those foods pro-inflammatory for them even though for the majority of people they are anti-inflammatory. See Chapter 1 for information on food allergies/intolerances and sensitivities. There are all types of good foods, but we will talk about some of the top ones.

1. **Ginger.** Herbalists have recommended the root of the ginger plant for thousands of years to help relieve tummy troubles. Not only does it help with the stomach, it contains natural anti-inflammatory effects and is used often as a common remedy for inflammation-related conditions. Ginger may help to calm arthritis pain by lowering hormone levels that induce inflammation. Some studies even suggest that ginger can reduce pain just as effectively as over-the-counter pain

relievers such as aspirin. Fresh ginger can be steeped in boiling water and used as a tea. You can try grating ginger in a dressing of extra virgin olive oil, lemon juice, minced garlic, and a little sea salt to top vegetables and salads. The mixture along with a little orange juice can make a great marinade for fish and meats as well. Grated ginger goes well with stir-fries and meat dishes, and is tasty in homemade baked goods. There are plenty of ways to include and enjoy ginger in your diet. Powdered capsule supplements are also available as well, but it is important to keep in mind that the supplement can act as a blood thinner, so let your doctor know if you plan to take this herb in supplement form.

2. **Turmeric.** Turmeric is an Indian spice that comes from the root of the *curcuma longa* plant, which is a relative to the ginger root. It is best known as a main ingredient in curry, but its deep yellow-orange color is also what gives ballpark mustard its bright yellow color. Turmeric has long been used in Chinese medicine as a powerful anti-inflammatory agent. The pigment that gives turmeric its yellow-orange color is called *curcumin*, and is believed to be the primary component of turmeric that contributes to its anti-inflammatory properties as well as its powerful antioxidant properties. Curcumin works by overpowering the pro-inflammatory proteins known as cytokines. Curcumin's anti-inflammatory effects have been shown to be comparable to the effects of potent prescription and over-the-counter anti-inflammatory medications and with no toxicity worries.

You can enjoy turmeric by using it in your daily meal plan. Try adding it to eggs, mixing it with brown rice, using it as a spice to flavor lentils or beans, adding it to salad dressing, adding it to certain vegetables, and even trying it in a smoothie. Turmeric is also available in powdered capsule form. The general recommendation is 400 to 600 mg, three times per day, of a standardized powder (curcumin). Be patient as it may take up to a few months before full benefits can take place. You shouldn't use turmeric supplements if you have gallstones or bile duct dysfunction. Speak with your doctor first before using a turmeric supplement if you have diabetes, are pregnant, are on blood thinning medications, and/or are on medication to reduce stomach acid.

3. **Tart cherries.** Cherries are the smallest member of the stone fruit family but they come with a big benefit. Cherries contain a very potent class of flavonoids called *anthocyanins*. Anthocyanins are what give cherries, berries, and other fruits and vegetables their deep rich colors. Cherries are an anthocyanin-rich food that delivers substantial antioxidant properties and anti-inflammatory activity, and can help to relieve pain by working in much the same way aspirin and nonsteroidal anti-inflammatory drugs do. Though both tart cherries and sweet cherries have high concentrations of anthocyanins, tart cherries (Balaton and Montmorency varieties) contain the highest content and also contain other supporting compounds. In addition, tart cherries are lower in sugar content than their sweet counterpart. You can eat cherries fresh, frozen, dried, or as cherry juice. Also, you can find tart cherry supplements in the form of capsules. Use as directed and discuss with your doctor. Cherries contain sorbitol and can trigger symptoms in those that have IBS and/or fructose malabsorption.

Your Nutrition Solution Tidbit

Flavonoids are plant pigments and the substance that gives fruits and vegetables their bright yellow, orange, and red colors. Flavonoids function as powerful antioxidants (protecting our body cells from damage that can lead to chronic disease) and provide tons of health benefits, including as an anti-inflammatory and as an antibiotic.

4. **Dark leafy greens.** Just about all vegetables contain a wide variety of phytonutrients, including flavonoids (quercitin) and carotenoids (lutein and beta-carotene), but dark green, leafy vegetables such as spinach, kale, and collard greens are at the top of the list in terms of their specific content. These specific veggies have more than a dozen different flavonoid compounds that function as anti-inflammatory and anti-cancer agents as well as antioxidants. Better yet, these veggies are chock-full of essential vitamins and minerals including vitamin E, vitamin C, vitamin K, vitamin A (in the form of carotenoids), folate, calcium, magnesium, iron and manganese, as well as fiber. You can enjoy dark leafy greens in salads (instead of your iceberg lettuce), in layers of lasagna, on sandwiches, steamed as a side dish, or chopped up in just about any casserole or soup.

5. **Nuts.** Who doesn't like a handful of walnuts, cashews, or almonds? But more than just tasting yummy, nuts are a great source of healthy inflammation-fighting nutrients and fats. Almonds in particular are rich in fiber, calcium, magnesium, potassium, and vitamin E whereas walnuts contain high levels of alpha-linolenic (ALA), a type of omega-3 fatty acid. All types of nuts

are packed with antioxidants that help the body fight off and repair damage caused by inflammation. Nuts are a major part of the Mediterranean diet. You can enjoy nuts in all types of ways, including as nut butters. But keep in mind, as healthy as they are, nuts contain fat, though a healthy fat, so a little bit packs in lots of calories. Therefore, watch your portion sizes.

Your Nutrition Solution Tidbit

Here is some good news! Many studies have concluded that cocoa powder and dark chocolate are full of antioxidant and anti-inflammatory properties.

---

6. **Green tea.** If coffee is your go-to beverage, consider making a change. Tea, especially green tea, is chock-full of potent antioxidant polyphenols that have anti-inflammatory properties. One particular antioxidant, called epigallocatechin-3-gallate (EGCG) and found in green and not black tea, may work to stop the production of certain inflammatory chemicals in the body as well as help to alleviate arthritis pain. One to three cups of green tea is recommended daily for these anti-inflammatory benefits. However, if you are caffeine sensitive, beware of caffeine content and choose a decaffeinated version.

7. **Ground flaxseed.** Some call it one of the most powerful plant foods on the planet. Flaxseeds are rich in omega-3 fatty acids, particularly in the form of linolenic acid (ALA). They are also rich in fiber, antioxidants, and lignans, which contain antioxidant and plant estrogen qualities. Both ALA and lignans may help to reduce

inflammation by blocking the release of certain pro-inflammatory compounds.

Ground flaxseed is much better absorbed than its whole counterpart. You can add about one to two tablespoons of ground flaxseed per day to your meal plan, but it's best not to use more than that. Flaxseed is usually not recommended during pregnancy. Add ground flaxseed to smoothies, non-fat yogurt, hot cereal, mashed potatoes, or in baked goods. Start small and increase slowly to avoid gastric upset.

8. **Extra-virgin olive oil.** Olive oil is a great anti-inflammatory, pain-busting monounsaturated fat to add to your daily meal plan. A compound found in extra-virgin olive oil specifically called *oleocanthal* acts similarly to that of non-steroidal anti-inflammatory drugs (NSAIDs) for warding off pain. Extra-virgin olive oil has stronger concentrations of phytonutrients than other olive oils, especially polyphenols, which have well-known and well-proven anti-inflammatory properties. Extra-virgin olive oil is the backbone of the Mediterranean diet due to its long list of health benefits, including lowering the risk for certain cancers, protecting against heart disease, and everything in between. Extra-virgin olive oil is the unrefined oil derived from the first pressing of the olives and is the olive oil that has the most delicate flavor. It can be drizzled on cooked veggies, used to sauté or brown foods, added to smoothies, used as a salad dressing, and used in baking.

9. **Raisins.** Raisins are probably not your first pick as a snack, but maybe they should be! Raisins are a dried up grape that can help keep inflammation in check. Raisins, along with other fruits, help to reduce the inflammation marker known as TNF-alpha. They are treated with

sulfur dioxide gas during processing to help preserve their color. Sulfur is one substance that is being explored for its role in joint health. In addition, these little wrinkled fruits contain anthocyanins, a class of polyphenolic antioxidants that have been found to have anti-inflammatory properties. Raisins are chock-full of vitamins, minerals, and all types of antioxidants.

10. **Salmon.** Salmon is a powerhouse food with amazing health benefits. Salmon and other fatty fish such as lake trout, sardines, herring, albacore tuna, and mackerel are a great source of lean, high-quality protein and contain no saturated fat. The type of fat they do provide is heart healthy omega-3 fatty acids in the form of EPA (eicosapentaenoic acid) and DHA (docosahexaenoic acid). These two powerful omega-3 fatty acids in fatty fish are good for your heart because they have anti-inflammatory properties. But they can also help fight inflammation in other parts of the body and help reduce pain by reducing the production of pro-inflammatory substances. The American Heart Association recommends two servings of fatty fish such as salmon per week for good heart health. Enjoy salmon and other varieties of fatty fish grilled, broiled, or baked. Substituting fish for high fat meats such as red meats can further aide in reducing chronic inflammation.

Your Nutrition Solution Tidbit

In addition to ginger and turmeric mentioned previously, there are quite a few other herbs and spices that can have anti-inflammatory effects and are worth adding to your regular cooking habits. These include cinnamon, garlic, cayenne, black pepper, rosemary, oregano, basil, clove, and nutmeg.

chapter 5

menu planning and shopping guide

Now that you have learned some essential tips on the best and healthiest way to eat for reducing inflammation, it is time to put that information to work by organizing weekly menus and grocery shopping. There will be times when sticking to your anti-inflammatory meal plan might get tricky, but this chapter will provide some helpful tips to get you through those times. Properly navigating the grocery store and mastering food labels will be two tools in your arsenal that will help you to choose foods that cause the least health issues and symptoms due to inflammation.

Menu Planning Tips

Controlling and preventing chronic inflammation means paying much closer attention to the foods that you purchase, prepare, and consume. Eating healthier, managing weight, exercising, and managing blood sugar are just some of the anti-inflammatory lifestyle changes that will have a big impact on your health. We have discussed all of these previously in the book, but here are a few additional tips to help you more easily plan your daily menus and be prepared for special circumstances.

- Get the family on board. It will be much easier to menu plan if others in your household are on board with this new, healthier way of eating. It will benefit the health of the entire family. Don't make one dish for yourself and another for the family. Explain to them the changes you will be making for your health and for theirs as well. The more they know and understand why changes are being made, the easier it will be on everyone.

- The best way to make changes in your diet is to plan ahead! Write out your menus for the week so that you are able to plan meals that avoid foods you should not have and include ones that you should. Your best bet is to cook at home and bring lunches to work or school until you get a handle on your new eating style. The more prepared you are, the less likely you will be to eat out, eat on the run, or grab something you shouldn't, all of which can spell trouble and make your anti-inflammatory eating style less effective. Once your weekly menus are planned, you can create your shopping list. This will help you to buy only what is on your list and not stray to foods you should be avoiding.

- Look for yummy new anti-inflammatory recipes to incorporate into your meal plan. Following an anti-inflammatory eating style is hardly a sacrifice. There are tons of fresh, healthy foods that fit into this type of eating style to explore and experience, and the easiest way to do that is to try new recipes. Look for anti-inflammatory, Mediterranean style, or Clean Eating recipes that will help you stick with your new way of eating and will still taste great.

- When planning both your meals and snacks, incorporate as many anti-inflammatory foods, spices, and herbs as possible, such as the ones we spoke about in Chapter 4. Choose a variety, especially of fruits and vegetables, to get a variety of essential vitamins, minerals, antioxidants, and phytonutrients. Keep this book and other resources handy while meal planning so you can go back and visit them when you have questions.

- Plan and be prepared for meals and snacks away from home. Don't put yourself in the situation to hit the drive-thru!

- Include a few meatless meals in your weekly meal plan. You will find them just as satisfying and you may find a few favorites.

- Avoid any of your own personal trigger foods, if you are aware of them. Don't assume that because a certain fruit or vegetable, for example, causes your joints to hurt a bit more, that you are intolerant to all fruits and vegetables. Keep a food diary so that you know which specific foods you need to stay away from and do not avoid whole food groups. A food diary is a good tool to help you create an anti-inflammatory eating plan that you will be able to implement long-term.

- Be creative and come up with some yummy substitutions in your menus for the foods that bother you the most so that you don't feel you are being deprived.

Your Nutrition Solution Tidbit

If you are not one to sit down and write things out, then grab your phone and find an app for that! There are plenty of apps out there for smartphones that can make meal planning and shopping lists easy and fun.

Make a Swap

Changing your diet for better health can sometimes feel like you have to give up everything you love to eat. It can be hard to give up some of the favorite foods that you were used to eating regularly. But the good news is that there is no need to feel deprived if you learn to make some smart and simple swaps that can lower calories, sugars, and unhealthy fats as well as help you avoid any specific foods that can generally or specifically trigger inflammation. These tips will get you started, but as you get used to your new eating approach, you will surely master the art of swapping.

Instead of:	Try:
Sugar	Cinnamon
Creamy salad dressings	Extra-virgin olive oil with vinegar and lemon juice
Mayonnaise	Pureed avocado or homemade guacamole
Cream pie	Greek yogurt, non-fat, and light, in the same flavor
Ice cream	Frozen yogurt topped with berries
Chocolate cake	Chocolate pudding, fat-free, sugar-free with light whipped topping

Milkshake	Smoothie made with soy milk, ground flaxseed, and any frozen fruit(s) of your choice
Soft drinks/soda	Green tea over ice, sweetened with a little honey and lemon
Cinnamon roll	Toasted whole grain English muffin, sprinkled with a touch of cinnamon
Apple pie	Fresh apple sprinkled with cinnamon and baked
Fast food french fries	Freshly cut potato (white or sweet potato), drizzled with olive oil and baked
Potato chips and dip	Homemade guacamole and raw veggies
Pizza	Homemade whole wheat pita bread, pizza sauce, part-skim mozzarella cheese, veggies
Burgers	Turkey burger (made of ground lean turkey breast) or a portabella mushroom brushed with extra-virgin olive oil and grilled. Try a lettuce wrap instead of a bun or use a thin whole grain sandwich bagel, add lettuce, tomato, onion, and other favorite veggie toppings.
Chili	Vegetarian chili. Make chili the way you normally would but add more beans, tomatoes, and other veggies such as corn and leave out the meat.

You get the idea! Whatever it is you like to eat, you *can* find a substitute that will be healthier and will be more anti-inflammatory than pro-inflammatory. It may take a little time to figure it out, but eventually you will be swapping foods like a champ and even enjoying it!

Dining Out

Just because you are following an anti-inflammatory eating plan doesn't mean you have to give up your social life of eating out with family and friends. It may be a little more challenging, but it can be done, and after you do it a few times, it will become second nature.

Here are a few tips to help you out:

- Plan ahead and make a mental note of what you might order depending on the restaurant you are going to. Many restaurants have their menu online so that you can check it out before you go and be prepared.

- Don't be afraid to ask your server questions or ask to have your food prepared a certain way. They are there to serve *you*!

- Most restaurant portion sizes are much larger than what you will need. Ask for a doggie bag when you order your meal and put half the entrée away before you begin to eat. That way you won't be tempted to over-indulge and eat the whole meal. Eating out too often can expand your waistline quickly.

- Avoid dishes with sauces and gravies, which can include loads of hidden unhealthy fats, sugars, dairy, and gluten as well as calories.

- Ask for substitutions. If your meal comes with french fries, ask for a salad, fresh fruit bowl, a plain baked potato or better yet, a sweet potato.

- If ordering a baked potato, leave off the butter and margarine and ask for a side of guacamole. It's great for chicken as well!

- Choose lean meats or fish that are not breaded and are broiled, baked, or grilled instead.

- Salad entrees make great choices, but watch your toppings. Stick with grilled chicken, turkey breast, shrimp, or lean ham. Add other healthier toppings such as avocado, beans, nuts, and seeds. Choose a variety of fresh veggies on top. Ask for plain extra-virgin olive oil or a vinaigrette as a salad dressing.

- When choosing sandwiches, opt for turkey breast, lean ham, or grilled chicken breast on whole grain bread, pita, wrap, or rolls. Top them with loads of veggies and use a healthier spread such as pureed avocado or guacamole instead of mayonnaise.

- Soups make great appetizers, side dishes, or even a main entrée. Choose healthy anti-inflammatory soups such as lentil, black bean, vegetable, butternut squash, or gazpacho.

Celebrating the Holidays

Holidays are always fun, but unfortunately they tend to center around lots and lots of food, no matter what the holiday! Because an anti-inflammatory diet is a permanent way of life, it's necessary to learn how to deal with holidays as they too are a part of normal life. It takes a little extra planning and preparation, but it will be well worth it for both your health and your holiday enjoyment.

- Plan in advance so that you can lessen your stress and anxiety concerning what to eat. This will allow you to more fully enjoy your holiday without amplifying your inflammation.

- Offer to host the family dinner so you have complete control over the food being served. It can make it much easier on you and your health in the long run.

- Don't forget to continue your exercise program. Holidays can be busy and stressful, so it's hardly the time to stop being active. Stress and inactivity can snowball into exacerbated symptoms, which is the last thing you need when you want to enjoy the holidays.

- Don't let the holidays expand your waist band. Keep food selection and portion sizes under control and don't use the holidays as an excuse to go wild. This is another good reason to keep up the exercise as well.

- Try healthier versions of your favorite holiday dishes. For example, add less sugar and use pureed fruit as a substitute for the fat in your pies. Make it fun to experiment and see just how healthy you can get those holiday dishes and still have them tasting fantastic. That is something to boast about! The Internet is a great place to start and you are surely to find recipes galore that fit your needs. Put your own spin on them and make them your holiday traditions.

- If you are not hosting the holiday get-together and going to friends or family, bring a few anti-inflammatory dishes and desserts to share. No one will know it is anti-inflammatory, and you'll know for sure that you'll have something to eat that won't cause problems for you.

- Don't avoid meals or snacks during the day to save up for a big holiday meal later! Continue to eat throughout the day as you normally would. Waiting until the big meal to eat can make it much more difficult to stick with the foods you know you should eat and to avoid the ones you shouldn't. Doing that can also wreak havoc on your blood sugar levels, which we know can be a trigger.

- You can try just about everything at the holiday meal, but take smaller portions so you don't overdo it and don't continue to do it night after night during the holidays. Don't make it a habit.

- Be careful not to consume too much alcohol, which can cause inflammation to rear its ugly head. Stick with a small glass or two of red wine and then switch to water with a lemon or lime.

Navigating the Supermarket

Consuming a diet that will help manage inflammation starts well before you sit down to eat. You need to be armed with a well-thought-out weekly meal plan and grocery list. Even with all of that in your arsenal, navigating your way through aisles and aisles of all types of foods can sometimes be overwhelming. Leave yourself plenty of time for grocery shopping so that you are able to shop wisely and knowledgeably. The goal is to stock your kitchen with healthy, wholesome foods that will fit into your anti-inflammatory meal plan. It's helpful to keep a running list of foods and beverages you need through the week so when you go to the grocery store you can stock up. Stocking your kitchen with healthy, anti-inflammatory foods will make it easier to stick to your new eating approach. It may take more time at first, but as you master the knowledge of what foods you can and can't have, grocery shopping will be a snap. Before you go shopping, make sure you eat a healthy meal or snack. Visiting the grocery store on an empty stomach can be your worst enemy!

Many of the larger chain stores allow you to create an on-line shopping list and offer guidelines and meal ideas for specific health conditions. In addition, many of the large chains now employ registered dietitians on the premises so if you get stuck on a food or have questions, don't be afraid to ask! That's what they are there for.

Grocery stores can be challenging with all of the foods you can and can't have staring you in the face at each turn. Your number one weapon should be a well-organized and well-thought-out grocery list that follows the menu plan you developed for the week. Here are a few tips to arm yourself with when you hit the grocery store so that you are able to fill your cart with the healthiest and most anti-inflammatory foods from each aisle.

Fruits and Vegetables Section

The first section to greet you in most grocery stores is the produce section that is full of all types and colors of fresh fruits and vegetables. This will be the largest section of the grocery store and the one you should spend most of your time in. Fruits and veggies make great healthy snacks and should be included with every meal. Fruits and vegetables are full of so many nutrients and phytochemicals that are your protection against inflammation. Fruit can even be a great substitution for sugary desserts when you have a sweet tooth. With so many types of fruits and vegetables available, you can't possibly come up with the excuse that you don't like them!

- Look for produce with the most color. The more colorful they are, the more nutrients and phyto- chemicals they contain. There are plenty to choose from, including broccoli, spinach, carrots, sweet potatoes, avocado, and red grapes, for example. But keep in mind that even white veggies such as on- ions and cauliflower contain loads of beneficial nu- trients too. In fact, onions contain a phytochemi- cal called *quercetin* that has anti-inflammatory and immune boosting properties and can help ease dis- comfort from arthritis as well as lower the risk of cancer, heart disease, and type 2 diabetes.

- Choose a variety of fruits and vegetables. Variety is the spice of life and the more variety you select the more nutritional value you will get in return. Be adventurous and try something new every week. You never know what you might find that you re- ally like.

- Buy fresh fruits and vegetables that are in season. You can always buy frozen when they are not in season. Opt for locally grown produce and organic when possible.

- Pre-cut fruits and vegetables can be very conve- nient for the busy person and family.

- When picking your fruits and vegetables, look them over carefully and choose the freshest ones.

- If buying canned fruit, choose ones that are canned in 100 percent juice and have no syrup added, which can add loads of refined sugar.

- If buying canned vegetables, select ones that are labeled "no salt" or "low sodium." Regular canned foods can be high in sodium.

- When buying fresh produce, buy only what you need so that you can eat it before it goes bad.

- Nuts and seeds are often found in this section of the grocery store and should be a part of your grocery list. They add healthy fats, fiber, and other nutritional value to your meal plan as well as having their own anti-inflammatory properties.

Dairy Section

The dairy section tends to line the perimeter of the grocery store. Even though it is usually labeled "the dairy case," it is filled with all types of foods, some in the dairy food group and some not. The dairy case usually includes foods such as milk and milk alternatives like soymilk, yogurts, cheeses, sour cream, cream cheese, eggs, puddings, butter and margarines, as well as hummus and other dips and spreads.

- Stick to low-fat and fat-free versions throughout the dairy case to lower your intake of unhealthy saturated fats.

- If using margarines or spreads, check the label for the words "partially hydrogenated" in the list of ingredients. These are the unhealthy trans fats and should be avoided at all cost! There are many margarine spreads that are now made without trans fats. Better yet, ditch the margarines, butters, etc. and stick with olive oil or nut butters.

- Choose yogurts that are fat-free or low-fat as well as "light." Greek yogurt is a great option because it provides more protein than regular yogurts.

- Although eggs are considered a protein choice, you can find eggs and egg white substitutes in this section as well. Egg white substitutes are a great alternative for whole eggs and a great way to lower your fat and cholesterol intake.

- Most importantly, if dairy is a food group that tends to bring on symptoms of inflammation for you, then learn how to swap these foods for others so that you do not miss the nutrients they provide. You can always swap regular milk for soy milk, almond milk, or rice milk. You can also try soy yogurt and soy cheese in place of their regular dairy counterparts. Check labels and ensure these foods are fortified especially with calcium and vitamin D, because we tend to get these nutrients mostly from milk products.

Meats/Seafood Section

The meat and seafood section is another area that is often found in the perimeter of the grocery store. This section includes fresh meats and seafood, as well as the deli section. Meats, especially red meats, can contain high amounts of unhealthy saturated fats, cholesterol, and plenty of pro-inflammatory substances. The goal here is to choose more lean meats and fish to help lower your risk for inflammation.

- Choose lean meat choices such as skinless white meat poultry, fish (wild caught), other seafood, pork loin, pork tenderloin, and ground turkey or chicken breast. Choose red meat only occasionally and select the leanest cuts, including top sirloin steak, eye of round roast or steak, top round roast and steak, flank steak, or extra lean ground beef (at least 90 percent or more lean). Cuts of meat are considered lean if they include the words "round" or "loin."

- If choosing beef, opt for grass-fed beef as opposed to grain fed. Grass-fed beef contains some omega-3 fatty acids, giving it a better ratio of omega-6 to omega-3 fats; contains slightly less saturated fat and twice as much CLA (conjugated linoleic acid) as grain fed, which is a fatty acid that is associated with some beneficial health effects.

- When it comes to deli meats, select lean turkey, roast beef, lean ham, or chicken breast and stay away from high saturated fat meats such as bologna and salami. Keep an eye on the sodium content and pick nitrate-free meats when possible.

- Choose fish as much as possible, especially fatty fish that contains more omega-3 fatty acids.

Breads/Cereal/Rice/Pasta Sections

As you get into the center aisles of the grocery store, you will encounter less fresh foods and more packaged and processed foods such as breads, cereals, rice, and pasta. These foods offer a great way to get your daily whole grain and fiber intake in, as well as other essential nutrients, if you make the right choices. Making the wrong choices in this section, on the other hand, can mean triggering inflammation, so choose wisely.

- Avoid refined foods such as white breads, regular pasta, white rice, and sugary cereals.

- Choose oatmeal, which is a hearty whole grain and high in fiber. Regular oatmeal is a better choice over instant because it is less processed. But even instant oatmeal is a whole grain and a better choice;

just watch the sugar content of flavored instant oatmeal. Flavor it yourself with cinnamon, raisins, or other fruits.

- When choosing dry cereals, select varieties that state "whole grain" and aim for at least four grams of fiber per serving. Read the label for sugar content as well and stick to ones that contain less than five grams of sugar per serving.

- Opt for whole wheat or whole grain breads. If it just states "wheat," it's not a whole grain product. Look back at Chapter 3 for more tips on choosing whole grains.

- Select whole grain foods such as brown or wild rice as opposed to white rice. Choose plain rice, as many of the packaged flavored rice are more processed and contain tons of sodium.

- Try alternate whole grains for something different such as bulgur, quinoa, barley, and whole grain couscous.

- Reading the food label is key in all sections, but especially in this one. You will need to read labels to ensure you are choosing foods that are truly whole grains and have the fiber content you expect without all of the sugar and sodium.

Canned Food Sections

The canned food section can include foods such as fruits, vegetables, tuna, beans, soups, and more. Keeping a variety of healthier canned goods on hand can ensure you always have something to reach for in a pinch. Choosing these foods, though not fresh, can still add plenty of nutrients to your required daily servings of certain foods groups. Canned foods can be just as nutritious if you make the right choices.

- Choose fruit that is canned in water or its own natural juices to keep the sugar content down. Stay away from ones that state "in syrup."
- Select vegetables that state "no salt" or "low sodium."
- Avoid buying canned vegetables that contain added fats such as sauces or butter as well as sodium. No need to ruin a good thing!
- Choose tuna or salmon that is packed in water, as opposed to packed in oils.
- Opt for lower fat and lower sodium soups and stick with the broth-based soups that contain loads of vegetables.
- Try beans such as black, kidney, lentils, garbanzo, and navy beans with no added salt to add to soups, casseroles, whole wheat pastas, and salads as an extra protein, nutrient, and fiber boost. Rinse canned beans to remove as much sodium as possible.

Oils, Condiments, and Dressings Section

This can be a dangerous section, as it is filled with foods that contain plenty of fat and sodium. It just takes making the right choices to get through this aisle in a healthy manner.

- Choose healthier oils such as extra virgin olive oil and canola oil. But whether healthy or not, use them sparingly. A little bit can go a long way and can pack in a lot of calories. Use them in place of unhealthier fats.

- Keep in mind that ketchup, salsa, and other condiments usually contain loads of sodium and may contain sugar as well. Select lower sugar and sodium versions or brands with the lowest amount of sugar and sodium per serving.

- Choose salad dressings that are more oil-based and are reduced-fat or light. Compare labels to pick brands that are lower in sodium and sugar. Your best choice for salad dressing is a little extra virgin olive oil with vinegar and a little lemon or lime juice.

- Try replacing regular mayonnaise with reduced-fat and fat-free versions or, better yet, for something more nutritious, substitute pureed avocado, guacamole, and hummus.

- Grab a can of fat-free cooking spray to use in sautéing and baking to save some additional calories.

Your Nutrition Solution Tidbit

When choosing olive oil, opt for extra virgin, which is the purest form of olive oil and the oil with the lowest acidity. This oil is great for dressings, drizzling on veggies, or brushing on breads. If you plan to cook with the oil, it's best to go with virgin or light olive oil as they are better suited for heat. Always check dates because oils have a limited shelf life and choose a bottle from the back of the shelf as light will tend to destroy the oil and its properties. Store it in a dark, cool, dry place once you get home.

Frozen Foods Section

The frozen food section entails a large variety of frozen foods such as vegetables, fruits, pizza, frozen entrees, breakfast foods like pancakes and waffles, specialty items, breads, juices, ice cream, and the list goes on. Frozen foods such as fruits and vegetables are a convenient way to always have produce on hand, especially during the winter months. Frozen foods can be convenient when you don't have time to cook, but just as in other sections of the grocery store, be sure to make the right choices.

- Read food labels in the freezer section. There are a wide variety of foods and you can always choose healthier options. For example, with frozen breakfast waffles, opt for the whole grain version.

- When choosing veggies, select ones that do not include sauces and butters. Many frozen vegetables come in ready-to-steam bags, which makes adding vegetables to meals even easier. Having frozen veggies on hand means you can always throw extra vegetables in soups, casseroles, pastas, and stews, or just add them as a side dish.

- Choose frozen fruit without added sugar. Frozen fruits are great for making smoothies, or adding to whole grain waffles for breakfast or to yogurt as a snack. Pick organic when possible.

- With frozen meals/entrees, always read the Nutrition Facts Panel first. These meals are fine on occasion when you don't have time to cook, but don't rely on them regularly. In general, look for meals that include plenty of vegetables, whole grains, lean meat, fish, or poultry. Skip ones that are sky high in carbs and ones that include cream sauces, gravies, or fried foods and are over 600 mg of sodium. Don't assume these meals are healthy without first checking the label.

Using Food Labels to Help Manage Inflammation

To truly follow an anti-inflammatory eating approach, you need to become a food label reader so that you can determine, without guessing, whether a food is healthy and whether it will fit within the guidelines of your meal plan. The food label is regulated by the FDA and is full of information including the Nutrition Facts Panel, Nutrient Content Claims, Health Claims, and Allergen information. Food labels are meant to be used by the consumer to compare foods and make better choices. They are especially helpful for those who are trying to follow a specific type of diet, but are really for everyone that wants to be more conscientious about what they eat.

The Nutrition Facts Panel

The Nutrition Facts Panel provides consumers with information about the nutrients that people should be most concerned with. This panel is the rectangular box on the back or side of packaged food and beverages that contains all of the nutritional information. The Nutrition Facts Panel was mandated under the Nutrition Labeling and Education Act (NLEA) of 1990 and is based on recommendations from the Food and Drug Administration (FDA) and the U.S. Department of Agriculture (USDA). Not only can this panel help you to manage both your overall health and inflammation, but your weight as well.

Nutrition Facts

Serving Size 1 cup (228g)
Servings Per Container about 2

Amount Per Serving

Calories 250	Calories from Fat 110

	% Daily Value*
Total Fat 12g	18%
Saturated Fat 3g	15%
Trans Fat 3g	
Cholesterol 30mg	10%
Sodium 470mg	20%
Total Carbohydrate 31g	10%
Dietary Fiber 0g	0%
Sugars 5g	
Proteins 5g	

Vitamin A	4%
Vitamin C	2%
Calcium	20%
Iron	4%

* Percent Daily Values are based on a 2,000 calorie diet.
Your Daily Values may be higher or lower depending on
your calorie needs:

		Calories:	2,000	2,500
Total Fat		Less than	65g	80g
Saturated Fat		Less than	20g	25g
Cholesterol		Less than	300mg	300mg
Sodium		Less than	2,400mg	2,400mg
Total Carbohydrate			300g	375g
Dietary Fiber			25g	30g

For educational purposes only. This label does not meet the labeling
requirements described in 21 CFR 101.9.

You can use the Nutrition Facts Panel to your advantage by following a few simple tips:

Sizing it Up

One of the initial parts of the label is the serving size, which is usually expressed in weight, volume, or number of units. Take a close look at the serving size and the servings per container.

- Ask yourself: How many calories are in a single serving? How many calories are in the entire package? How many servings do I plan to eat?

- All of the nutrition information on the Nutrition Facts Panel pertains to that one specified single serving size. Simply looking at the nutrition information won't mean much if you don't pay attention to the serving size.

- If you plan on eating two servings, then you need to double *all* of the information, including calories, nutrients, and fat.

- When comparing calories and nutrients on the same food but between brands, check to see if the serving size is the same.

Your Nutrition Solution Tidbit

Many food packages, and that includes beverages, contain more than one serving. Don't fall into the trap of assuming there is only one serving in a package and consuming the whole package before you read the label first. That can add up to a lot more carbs, calories, and fat than you planned on.

Focusing on Calories

Next on the label are calories and calories from fat. This is important for determining whether a food is appropriate for your meal plan, especially if you are trying to lose weight. High fat foods can mean more calories and, with time, weight gain.

- Whether you are focusing on losing weight or maintaining a healthy weight, keep in mind that just because foods are fat free does not make them calorie free! Foods void of fats are many times high in sugar and contain plenty of calories.

- Check to see how many total calories the food contains and how many of those calories come from fat. For example, if a food has 300 calories per serving and 150 of those calories come from fat, then half of the calories in a single serving come from a fat source.

- Consider how the calories per serving will fit into your total calorie goal for the day. The key is to keep your calories in check as you lose or manage your weight. Keep in mind that if you eat and drink more calories than you burn, you *will* gain weight and in turn you will increase your risk for inflammation.

- In general, you can use this guide to gauge the calories in a single product (based on a 2,000-calorie diet). But when it comes to body weight, what really matters is the total calories you consume in a day and not what is in a single food:
  - ◉ LOW in calories = 40 calories per serving
  - ◉ MODERATE in calories = 100 calories per serving
  - ◉ HIGH in calories = 400 calories or more per serving

Limiting These Nutrients

The nutrients listed first on the label are the ones that most Americans generally consume enough or too much of in their diet. Nutrients to limit for better health and a lower risk of inflammation include total fat, saturated fat, trans fat, cholesterol, and sodium. Not only is it important to know how much total fat is in a serving of a food, but what type of fat it is. Saturated and trans fats are the ones you want to limit and keep as low as possible because we know they can trigger inflammation as well as other health issues. On the other hand, fats that you want to include are monounsaturated and polyunsaturated fats as they are healthy fats and can lower the risk for inflammation as well as other health conditions.

Getting Enough of These Nutrients

The nutrients listed next on the label are those that most Americans don't get enough of but need in their daily diet. These include dietary fiber, vitamin A, vitamin C, calcium, and iron. Eating enough of these nutrients can help improve health and reduce the risk of some health conditions and diseases. Eating a diet high in fiber promotes anti-inflammation and blood sugar control and can help with weight loss and/or maintenance.

Figuring Out Percent Daily Value

If you are not sure whether a food is high or low in the nutrients mentioned previously, the Percent Daily Value (%DV) is a tool on the label that can help you figure that out. Start with the footnote on the bottom of the label, which tells you that %DVs are based on a 2,000-calorie diet. This statement must appear on all food labels. This part of the food label is the same on *all* labels and does not change from product to product like the rest of the information. This information is recommended dietary advice for all Americans and is not specific to the food product.

	Calories:	2,000	2,500
Total Fat	Less than	65g	80g
Sat Fat	Less than	20g	25g
Cholesterol	Less than	300mg	300mg
Sodium	Less than	2,400mg	2,400mg
Total Carbohydrate		300g	375g
Dietary Fiber		25g	30g

*Percent Daily Values are based on a 2,000 calorie diet. Your Daily Values may be higher or lower depending on your calorie needs.

The recommendations for total fat, saturated fat, carbohydrates, and fiber are all based on a 2,000-calorie diet. If you eat less than or more than the calorie levels used, you need to adjust the recommended dietary advice to fit your individual needs. Cholesterol and sodium recommendations are the same no matter what calorie level you are consuming. The following is a chart of how the Percent Daily Values need to be adjusted according to calorie level:

Adjusted Percent Daily Values for Specific Calorie Levels	
Calories	**Adjusted %DV**
1,200	60 percent
1,400	70 percent
1,600	80 percent
2,000	100 percent
2,200	110 percent
2,500	125 percent
2,800	140 percent
3,200	160 percent

Putting %DV to Use

Now that you know what the Daily Values are, we can use them to determine Percent Daily Value (%DV), which will help you decide whether a food is high or low in a nutrient and, ultimately, if it is a smart food to choose. The %DV is listed to the right of most of the nutrients on the top part of the label.

To help you decide quickly, use this guide:

5% DV or less is considered LOW for that nutrient.

20% DV or more is considered HIGH for that nutrient.

Get enough of these nutrients. The goal is to stay above 100% DV for each of these for the entire day:

- Fiber.
- Vitamin A.
- Vitamin C.
- Calcium.
- Iron.

Limit the following nutrients. The goal is to stay below 100% DV for each of these for the entire day:

- Total fat. (Stick to mostly polyunsaturated and monounsaturated fats, which are healthier fats.)
- Saturated fat.
- Cholesterol.
- Sodium.

You can use %DV not only to figure out if a food is high or low in a nutrient, but also to compare products. You can easily compare one product or brand to a similar product to make the better choice. Just make sure that when you compare, the serving sizes are similar. Serving sizes are kept generally consistent for similar types of foods to make comparing them easier for the consumer.

You can also use %DV to help you make dietary trade-offs with other foods throughout the day. This allows you to eat all of your favorite foods, on occasion, and fit them into a healthy anti-inflammatory diet. For instance, when one of your favorite foods is high in fat, you can balance it with foods that are lower in fat at other times of the day. But pay attention to how much you eat of that favorite food so that the total amount of fat for your day stays below the 100% DV.

One more way to use %DV is to help you distinguish one dietary claim from another such as "light" versus "reduced fat." All you need to do is compare the %DVs for total fat in each of the foods to determine which one is higher or lower in that nutrient. This way, there is no need to memorize all of the definitions that go along with those claims.

Additional Nutrient Information

The label also provides %DVs for a few vitamins and minerals, including Vitamins A and C, calcium, and iron. You may see more on some labels, but you will at minimum always see these four nutrients. Use the %DV given so that you know how much one serving of a food contributes to the total amount you need per day.

The Daily Values used for these four nutrients are as follows:

- Vitamin A: 5,000 IU
- Vitamin C: 60 mg
- Calcium: 1,000 mg
- Iron: 18 mg

Note: For certain populations, some of these numbers may be higher or lower; these are general values.

For example, if calcium is listed as 25% DV, then one serving of that food will provide you with 25 percent of what you need for the day or 250 mg.

Always check labels and don't make assumptions. Just because yogurt is supposed to be a good calcium source doesn't mean it is the same in every yogurt. Before you buy, compare brands and choose the ones that have the most calcium and protein and the lowest sugar and fat content. Use the nutrition labels! They are on food products for the consumers' use!

Your Nutrition Solution Tidbit

The %DV for trans fat, sugar, and protein have not yet been established. However, you can still compare total amounts between brands to pick the better product.

Putting It All Together

Once you have checked out all parts of the food label, you need to ask yourself if this particular food is a smart choice. Does it fit into a healthy diet, into your weight management plan and, most importantly, does it fall into the anti-inflammatory category? Ask these questions to find out:

- Is one serving size enough for me or do I need to double, triple, etc. the carbs, calories, fat, and other nutrients on the label?
- Are the calories per serving low, moderate, or high? How many calories will be in the actual amount I eat?

- Are the nutrients that I need to limit low and are the nutrients I need more of high? Are there plenty of anti-inflammatory nutrients for this product to be worth it?

- Is this food too high in fat, especially saturated and trans fat?

- Does this food contain sugar or too much sugar for my needs?

- Will this food provide me with some needed fiber?

- Have I compared the label on this product to other brands of the same to ensure I am getting the most bang for my buck? Should I look for an alternative?

How you answer these questions will differ from one person to the next depending on your calorie intake; whether you are trying to lose, maintain, or gain weight; whether you might have specific nutritional needs; if you have specific health issues; and how critical your inflammation has become. The bottom line is that food labels enable you to compare foods based on key ingredients and, therefore, make better choices for your anti-inflammatory meal plan. Food labels allow you to include your favorite foods occasionally, even if they are not always the smartest choices, but still stick to your healthy eating plan and goals. Use the Nutrition Facts Panel to make your food choices easier and healthier!

Nutrient Content Claims

Even if you don't have time to read each and every food label, something known as "Nutrient Content Claims" can help you to quickly find foods that meet your specific needs and goals. The definition, by the FDA, of a nutrient content claim on a food product directly or by implication characterizes the level of a nutrient in a food such as "low-fat," "fat-free," "high in fiber," or "reduced sugar." Each and every claim that is used on food packaging has a very specific definition. These are a few of the more popular ones that are used on food labels:

- **Reduced or Less** means at least 25 percent less calories, total fat, saturated fat, sugar, sodium, or cholesterol than the regular product. This might not necessarily mean the product is "low" in a nutrient if the regular product is quite high.

- **Light or Lite** means the food contains one third fewer calories or no more than half the fat of the regular or higher-calorie, higher-fat version, or no more than half the sodium of the higher sodium version.

- **Good Source, Contains, or Provides** means the food contains between 10 to 19 percent of the daily value for a nutrient per serving.

- **Excellent Source of, High, Rich in** means the food contains 20 percent or more of the daily value for a nutrient per serving.

- **More, Fortified, Enriched, Added, Extra, or Plus** means the food contains 10 percent or more of the daily value for a nutrient per serving compared to the regular product.

- **No Added Sugars** means no sugar or sugar-containing ingredient is added during processing.

- **Sugar-free** means less than 0.5 grams of sugar per serving.

- **Low-fat** means three grams of fat or less per serving.

- **Fat-free** means less than 0.5 grams of fat per serving.

- **Cholesterol-free** mean less than two milligrams of cholesterol and two grams or less of saturated fat per serving.

- **Low-sodium** means 140 mg or less of sodium per serving.

- **Sodium-free** means less than five milligrams of sodium per serving.

- **Low-calorie** means 40 calories or less per serving.

- **Calorie-free** means less than five calories per serving.

- **Lean (on meat labels)** means less than 10 grams of fat per serving, with 4.5 grams or less of saturated fat, and 95 milligrams of cholesterol per serving.

- **Extra Lean (on meat labels)** means less than five grams of fat per serving, with less than two grams of saturated fat, and 95 milligrams of cholesterol.

Health Claims

Health claims on labels are another tool to help you make healthier choices that are individualized to you and your specific health issues. The definition, by the FDA, of a health claim means any claim made on the label or in the labeling of a food, including dietary supplements, that expressly or by implication, including "third party" references, written statements, symbols, or vignettes, characterizes the relationship of any substance to a disease or health-related condition. Implied health claims include those statements, symbols, vignettes, or other forms of communication that suggest, within the context in which they are presented, that a relationship exists between the presence or level of a substance in the food and a disease or health-related condition.

Some examples of just a few health claims include:

- "Diets rich in whole grain foods and other plant foods and low in total fat, saturated fat, and cholesterol may help reduce the risk of heart disease."
- "Low fat diets rich in fiber-containing grain products, fruits, and vegetables may reduce the risk of some types of cancer, a disease associated with many factors."
- "Low fat diets rich in fiber-containing grain products, fruits, and vegetables may reduce the risk of some types of cancer, a disease associated with many factors."

Note: To find all of the nutrient content claims and health claims, visit the FDA at www.fda.gov.

Allergen Listings

Because inflammatory triggers can be due to high allergen foods, it is important to know that you can use food labels to detect whether a food contains a specific ingredient that you might be allergic or sensitive to. In the U.S., the FDA requires manufacturers to list the eight most common ingredients that can trigger food allergies under the Food Allergen Labeling and Consumer Protection Act (FALCPA).

The eight foods that are included in food allergy labeling include:

- Milk.
- Egg.
- Fish.
- Crustacean shellfish.
- Tree nuts.

- Wheat.
- Peanuts.
- Soybeans.

Labels list the type of allergen, for example, tree nut (almond) or the type of shellfish, such as crab or shrimp. Also listed are any ingredients that contain a protein from the eight major food allergens as well as any allergens found in flavorings, colorings, and other additives. The Food Allergen Labeling law requires food allergens to be specified on the label no matter what the quantity, but only when they are contained as an ingredient.

Your Nutrition Solution Tidbit

Manufacturers are *not* required to include warnings concerning food allergens and cross-contamination or food allergens accidently being introduced during manufacturing or packaging. This can be trouble if you are very sensitive to a food allergen. However, many manufacturers tend to include warnings voluntarily, though not always in a clear manner. The FDA is working to make this more consistent so that it is easier for consumers to identify allergens with no worries. If you are in doubt and you do have an allergy or sensitivity, call the manufacturer and/or check with your doctor.

Although gluten is not on the list of major allergens and it is really not considered a food allergy, there are many people that are intolerant of gluten or have celiac disease, a chronic digestive disorder, and cannot consume any amount of gluten. In addition, there are those people who experience inflammatory triggers from consuming gluten. Gluten is a protein found in wheat, barley, and rye, and is found in many foods and food ingredients. The good news is that the FDA has established a ruling defining guidelines for the use of the term "gluten-free" on packaged food labels. This will greatly help those who need to live gluten-free to be confident that items labeled "gluten-free" meet a defined standard for gluten content. The new ruling states that any food labeled "gluten-free" contain less than 20 parts per million of the protein.

The bottom line is that if you have food allergies or sensitivities that you know are inflammatory triggers for you, then be aware of what you are eating and drinking and be sure to check labels. Even if a food may have been safe to eat the last time you bought it, check again because manufacturers change their ingredients often. If you have any doubt, contact the manufacturer about whether the food possibly contains a specific allergen, including gluten.

chapter 6

14-day menu guide and stocking your kitchen

To this point you have been provided with a great deal of information that will help you start using nutrition as a large part of managing chronic inflammation. This chapter will help you put it all together by providing 14 days of easy-to-follow menus to get you started on the right foot. You can use these menus as a beginning point to plan your own menus with your individual likes and dislikes. In addition, this chapter will provide you with an extensive list of all the foods and beverages that are great to have on hand in your kitchen to keep inflammation in check.

14-Day Menu Guide

The following menus are chock-full of anti-inflammatory foods and void of the foods that are commonly considered pro-inflammatory. As you become more familiar with which foods are best, you can venture out to recipes, which you will find tons of on the Internet! Portion sizes will need to be adjusted depending on your individual caloric need and your weight loss/maintenance goals. The menus are low in saturated, trans fat, cholesterol, refined sugars, and moderate in sodium. They include great sources of omega-3 fatty acids and monounsaturated fats. In addition, they provide plenty of fiber and anti-inflammatory nutrients. You will need to substitute any foods included in the menus that are personal trigger foods for you. The format of these menus follow the recommendation of frequent and smaller meals for plenty of opportunities to get your food groups in, keep your hunger satisfied, and keep your metabolism burning throughout day. If you get hungry after dinner, snack on fruit, yogurt, nuts, seeds, light popcorn, whole grain crackers, etc. Don't forget to drink plenty of water throughout the day as well.

Your Nutrition Solution Tidbit

Don't forget your water intake throughout the day. Staying hydrated is essential for good health and just about every function in your body. In addition, water is important for keeping joints properly lubricated, so if you deal with arthritis, then water is especially helpful.

Day 1

Breakfast

Steel-cut oatmeal, cooked with water, topped with raspberries, sliced almonds, cinnamon, light soymilk
Green tea.

<u>A.M. Snack</u>

Apple slices dipped in almond butter

<u>Lunch</u>

Wrap: chicken breast, skinless, cooked, diced; mashed avocado, baby spinach leaves; and diced tomato in whole wheat tortilla or whole wheat pita.

Grapes, seedless, red or green

Sliced strawberries

<u>P.M. Snack</u>

Goat cheese spread on whole wheat crackers

Ginger tea*

<u>Dinner</u>

Salmon, wild-caught, grilled or baked (marinate with lite teriyaki sauce, extra virgin olive oil, and a few shakes of ground ginger for a few hours before cooking).

Asparagus, fresh, steamed, drizzle with extra virgin olive oil.

Brown rice mixed with a few shakes of ground turmeric.

Day 2

<u>Breakfast</u>

English muffin, whole grain, toasted, spread with almond butter

Cantaloupe, cubed

Turkey sausage links, cooked

Soymilk, light

Ginger tea*

A.M. Snack

Greek yogurt, non-fat, mix in 1 Tbs. ground flaxseed and blueberries

Lunch

Sandwich: fresh turkey breast or nitrate-free deli meat with mashed avocado or guacamole, spinach leaves, sliced tomato in whole wheat pita.

Baby carrots

Celery stalks, trimmed

P.M. Snack

Grapes, seedless, red or green

Almond milk

Dinner

Skinless chicken breast, baked, broiled or grilled

Broccoli, steamed

Sweet potato, baked with 1 Tbs. non-trans fat margarine

Dark green leafy salad topped with extra virgin olive oil, balsamic vinegar, and a dash of lemon and pinch of ground turmeric.

Green tea

Day 3

Breakfast

Bran cereal topped with blueberries and fat-free milk
Ginger tea*

A.M. Snack

Low-fat cottage cheese topped with ground cinnamon
and sliced peaches

Lunch

Romaine lettuce with fresh veggies such as red peppers,
broccoli, and cucumber, topped with garbanzo beans,
sunflower seeds, chopped egg whites, and extra-virgin
olive oil, balsamic vinegar, and a pinch of ground turmeric as dressing.

P.M. Snack

Hummus and baby carrots or celery sticks

Dinner

Stir-fry of shrimp, edamame, red pepper, onion, water
chestnuts, ground or grated ginger, soy sauce, minced
garlic, and extra virgin olive oil
Serve over cooked brown rice or whole grain couscous

Day 4

Breakfast

Steel-cut oatmeal, cooked with water, topped with ground cinnamon and raisins

Pear

Soymilk, light

Green tea

A.M. Snack

Smoothie made with banana, sliced strawberries, and soymilk, light and 1 Tbs. ground flaxseed (you can use frozen fruit to make the smoothie thicker and can add protein powder, optional).

Lunch

Tuna salad wrap: 3 oz. tuna, canned in water, mixed with 1 1/2 Tbs. non-fat Greek yogurt, 1 1/2 Tbs. mashed avocado, 1 Tbs. diced celery, 1 tsp. Dijon mustard and garlic powder to taste. Roll tuna salad in whole wheat tortilla.

Vegetable soup, low sodium

1 apple

P.M. Snack

Guacamole (for a twist, try adding quinoa to your guacamole)

Fresh veggies for dipping

Ginger tea*

<u>Dinner</u>

Mix together:

- 1 1/2 cups pasta, whole wheat, cooked.
- 1/2 cup black beans, canned, drained.
- 1/2 cup carrots, steamed.
- 1/4 cup peas, steamed.
- 1/2 cup zucchini, steamed.
- 1/2 Tbs. extra virgin olive oil plus 2 Tbs. freshly grated Parmesan cheese.

Dark green leafy salad greens with raw vegetables, topped with extra virgin olive oil plus balsamic vinegar with a bit of lemon juice and pinch of ground turmeric.

Day 5

<u>Breakfast</u>

Whole grain bagel topped with almond nut butter

Sliced strawberries

Ginger tea*

<u>A.M. Snack</u>

Smoothie made with blackberries and soymilk, light and 1 Tbs. ground flaxseed. (You can use frozen fruit to make the smoothie thicker and can add optional protein powder.)

Lunch

Veggie wrap: diced tomato, baby spinach, black beans, and diced avocado wrapped in a whole wheat tortilla

Celery and carrot sticks

Orange

P.M. Snack

Handful of cashews and raisins

Dinner

Skinless chicken breast marinated in lemon and ground turmeric, grilled or baked

Wild rice, cooked

Zucchini, steamed

Day 6

Breakfast

Whole grain waffle topped with peanut butter

Cantaloupe, cubed

Orange juice, 100 percent juice, calcium fortified

A.M. Snack

Handful of walnuts

1 grapefruit

Green tea

Lunch

Soup, lentil, low sodium (sprinkle in a little ground turmeric)

6 whole wheat crackers

1 pear

P.M. Snack

Popcorn, plain, light

Dinner

Salmon, wild caught, broiled, baked, or grilled (marinate it ahead of time with soy sauce, extra virgin olive oil, and sprinkle with ginger and garlic).

Whole grain couscous, cooked and mixed with salsa and black beans

Spinach, steamed

Day 7

Breakfast

Egg whites scrambled with fresh sliced mushrooms, diced tomatoes and chopped spinach

Whole grain bagel topped with almond butter

Strawberries, sliced

Ginger tea*

A.M. Snack

Apple spread with peanut butter

<u>Lunch</u>

Skinless chicken breast, cooked, diced, wrapped in whole wheat tortilla with black beans, diced tomato, sliced avocado, and salsa.

Cottage cheese, low-fat, sprinkled with ground cinnamon and topped with peaches.

<u>P.M. Snack</u>

Hummus

Fresh veggies for dipping

<u>Dinner</u>

Extra lean ground turkey breast burger on whole grain pita topped with sliced avocado, sliced tomato, and spinach leaves.

Dark green leafy salad with raw vegetables, topped with extra virgin olive oil plus balsamic vinegar, lemon, and a pinch of ground turmeric.

Day 8

<u>Breakfast</u>

Steel-cut oatmeal, cooked, topped with ground cinnamon, chopped walnuts, blueberries

Soymilk, light

Grapefruit

A.M. Snack

Smoothie. Mix together in blender:

- 1 banana.
- 1/2 cup Greek yogurt, non-fat, plain.
- 1 cup soymilk, light.
- 1 Tbs. honey.
- 1/4 tsp. ginger root, grated finely.
- 1/4 cup ice.

Lunch

Black bean soup, low sodium
Whole grain crackers
Cantaloupe, diced

P.M. Snack

Handful of almonds and raisins

Dinner

Halibut, baked, sprinkle with garlic
Roasted butternut squash, drizzle with cinnamon and extra virgin olive oil
Broccoli, steamed

Day 9

<u>Breakfast</u>

Whole grain English muffin topped with almond butter

Canadian bacon or turkey bacon, cooked

Hard-boiled egg

Cantaloupe, diced

<u>A.M. Snack</u>

Greek Yogurt, non-fat mixed with 1 Tbs. ground flax-seed and pinch of ground cinnamon

Ginger tea*

<u>Lunch</u>

3 oz. tuna, canned in water mixed with 1 1/2 Tbs. Greek yogurt, non-fat, 1 1/2 Tbs. mashed avocado, 1 Tbs. diced celery, 1 tsp. Dijon mustard and garlic powder to taste

Spread on whole grain crackers

Lentil soup, low sodium

Ginger tea*

<u>P.M. Snack</u>

Popcorn, light

Apple

Green tea

Dinner

Skinless, chicken breast, grilled

Sautéed mushrooms and zucchini, in extra virgin olive oil and minced garlic mixed into whole grain spaghetti noodles, cooked, sprinkled with fresh parmesan cheese.

Romaine salad with fresh veggies, topped with extra virgin olive oil, vinegar, lemon, and a pinch of ground turmeric.

Day 10

Breakfast

Bran cereal with fat-free milk and sliced strawberries

Orange juice, 100 percent juice, calcium fortified

Ginger tea*

A.M. Snack

Handful of raisins and walnuts

Tart cherries

Lunch

Hard-boiled egg

Cottage cheese topped with blueberries and sprinkled with ground cinnamon

Green tea

<u>P.M. Snack</u>

Smoothie. Mix together in blender:

- 1/2 cup blackberries, frozen.
- 1/2 cup Greek yogurt, non-fat, plain.
- 1 cup soymilk, light.
- 1 Tbs. honey.
- 1/4 tsp. ginger root, grated finely.

<u>Dinner</u>

Trout, baked
Cauliflower, steamed and sprinkled with turmeric
Spinach, steamed
Sweet potato, baked with non-trans fat margarine

Day 11

<u>Breakfast</u>

Cooked quinoa topped with ground cinnamon, blueberries, and walnuts
Soymilk, light
Green tea

<u>A.M. Snack</u>

Smoothie made with:

- Banana.
- Sliced strawberries.
- Almond milk.

- 1 Tbs. ground flaxseed.

(You can use frozen fruit to make the smoothie thicker and can add optional protein powder.)

<u>Lunch</u>

Romaine lettuce salad with fresh veggies such as broccoli, red onions, and cucumber, topped with garbanzo beans, pumpkin seeds, chopped egg whites, and extra virgin olive oil, balsamic vinegar, lemon juice with a pinch of turmeric as a dressing.

Green tea

<u>P.M. Snack</u>

Hummus

Raw broccoli and cauliflower

Ginger tea*

<u>Dinner</u>

Turkey kielbasa, baked, broiled, or grilled

Bun, whole grain

1 tsp. Dijon mustard

Sweet potato, homemade french fries, oven baked

1 cup broccoli, steamed

Day 12

<u>Breakfast</u>

Breakfast sandwich: egg whites, scrambled; goat cheese, Canadian bacon, cooked; English muffin, whole grain, toasted

Grapefruit

Ginger tea*

<u>A.M. Snack</u>

Apple spread with almond butter

<u>Lunch</u>

Vegetable and barley soup, low sodium (add some curry powder for a little heat).

Dark green leafy salad with fresh veggies, topped with extra virgin olive oil, vinegar, lemon, ground turmeric.

<u>P.M. Snack</u>

Trail mix: almonds, dried pineapple, raisins

<u>Dinner</u>

Turkey meatballs, made with extra lean turkey breast

Spaghetti, whole grain

Spaghetti sauce, homemade

Dark green leafy salad with fresh veggies, topped with extra-virgin olive oil, vinegar, lemon, ground turmeric.

Day 13

Breakfast

Cooked quinoa topped with ground cinnamon and blackberries
Almond milk
Ginger tea*

A.M. Snack

Rice cakes, brown rice topped with almond butter
Grapes, seedless, red or white

Lunch

Barley salad: start with cooked barley and add your favorite cooked veggies, beans, and even tofu.
Green tea

P.M. Snack

Tart cherries
Walnuts

Dinner

Pork tenderloin, baked or grilled
Oven-steamed spaghetti squash, drizzle with extra virgin olive oil
Zucchini, steamed

Day 14

Breakfast

Whole grain English muffin with almond butter and honey

Grapefruit

Ginger tea*

A.M. Snack

Greek or Soy yogurt, non-fat with 1 Tbs. flaxseed and mixed berries (Eat as is or use frozen mixed berries and blend for a smoothie.)

Lunch

Chili made with kidney beans, onion, tomato sauce, corn, extra-lean ground turkey, and whatever else you want to add! Put in a pinch of turmeric, garlic, and other spices. Add curry if you want to spice it up.

Dark green leafy salad with fresh veggies, topped with extra virgin olive oil, vinegar, lemon, and ground turmeric.

P.M. Snack

Brown rice, rice cakes topped with almond butter

Walnuts

Dinner

Salmon, grilled or baked, topped with mango salsa

Fresh asparagus, steamed

Cauliflower, steamed

To make ginger tea: grate about 1/4 inch fresh ginger and allow to steep in hot water for about 10 minutes. You can add natural sweetener such as agave nectar or honey.

Stocking Your Kitchen

A well-stocked kitchen with plenty of anti-inflammatory, healthy foods will make life much easier. When you know you can grab a snack or a quick meal with the foods you have in your kitchen, you will relieve some of the stress and anxiety about managing inflammation. You might find that your whole family will eat healthier once you have your kitchen stocked properly. This is only a sampling of foods to get you started. Of course, there are many more you can add; just make sure they are on the safe list, as well as the healthy list. Keep in mind that you may need to adjust this list for any foods that you are allergic or sensitive to, or foods that you find cause trouble. This is far from an extensive list of foods that are healthy and safe in an anti-inflammatory diet, but it gives you a good starting point.

Fruits (Fresh, frozen, or canned in its own juice; organic when possible.)

- Apples.
- Apricots.
- Avocados.
- Bananas.
- Blackberries.
- Blueberries.
- Cantaloupe.
- Cherries (especially tart cherries).
- Cranberries.

- Prunes.
- Grapefruit.
- Grapes.
- Kiwi.
- Lemons.
- Limes.
- Mangoes.
- Oranges.
- Peaches.
- Pears.
- Pineapples.
- Plums.
- Raisins.
- Raspberries.
- Strawberries.
- Watermelon.

Vegetables (Fresh, frozen, or canned with low or no salt; organic when possible.)

- Asparagus.
- Beets.
- Bell peppers (green, red, orange, and yellow).
- Broccoli.
- Brussel sprouts.
- Cabbage (red or green).
- Carrots.
- Cauliflower.
- Celery.
- Corn.

- Green beans.
- Kale.
- Mushrooms.
- Onions.
- Peas.
- Potatoes.
- Radishes.
- Romaine lettuce.
- Scallions.
- Spinach.
- Squash (summer or winter).
- Sweet potatoes.
- Swiss chard.
- Tomatoes.
- Zucchini.

Grains
- Amaranth.
- Barley.
- Brown rice.
- Buckwheat.
- Bulgur.
- Kamut.
- Millet.
- Oatmeal (old fashioned or steel cut).
- Popcorn (light).
- Quinoa.
- Spelt.

- Wheat berries.
- Whole grain/wheat breads, pitas, tortillas, rolls, etc.
- Whole wheat pasta.
- Whole grain crackers.
- Wild rice.

Fish and Shellfish (Freeze it until needed.)

- Cod.
- Flounder.
- Halibut.
- Mackerel.
- Mussels.
- Oysters.
- Salmon (wild).
- Sardines (canned in olive oil or water).
- Shrimp.
- Trout.
- Tuna (canned in water).

Proteins and Meats (Grass-fed when possible; freeze until needed.)

- Skinless chicken breast.
- Skinless turkey breast.
- Ground turkey breast.
- Pork tenderloin.
- Tofu.
- Tempeh.
- Eggs/egg whites.

Dairy Products

- Soymilk, light.
- Almond milk.
- Rice milk.
- Fat-free milk.
- Greek yogurt, non-fat, light.

Herbs and Spices (Fresh or dried)

- Allspice.
- Basil.
- Bay leaf.
- Cilantro.
- Cinnamon.
- Curry powder.
- Clove.
- Dill.
- Garlic.
- Ginger.
- Marjoram.
- Mustard.
- Nutmeg.
- Paprika.
- Parsley.
- Pepper (black or red).
- Peppermint.
- Rosemary.
- Saffron.
- Sage.
- Tarragon.

- Thyme.
- Turmeric.

Legumes, Nuts, and Seeds

- Almonds.
- Black beans.
- Cashews.
- Chia Seeds.
- Garbanzo beans (chickpeas).
- Ground flaxseed.
- Kidney beans.
- Lentils.
- Navy beans.
- Peanuts.
- Pine nuts.
- Pinto beans.
- Pumpkin seeds.
- Sesame seeds.
- Soybeans/edamame.
- Split peas.
- Sunflower seeds.
- Walnuts.

Oils/Fats

- Extra virgin olive oil.
- Canola oil.
- Evening primrose oil.
- Walnut oil.
- Grapeseed oil.

- Nut butters (such as almond butter).
- Peanut butter.

Miscellaneous Items

- Dark chocolate, plain.
- Honey.
- Green tea.
- Red wine.
- Apple cider vinegar.
- Guacamole.
- Hummus.

your best resources

Websites

Arthritis Foundation: *www.arthritis.org.*

Georgia State University Center for Inflammation, Immunity and Infection: *http://inflammation.gsu.edu/ about-the-center/research-facilities-and-resources-center-for-inflammation-immunity-infection-georgia-state-university/.*

Center for Human Immunology, Autoimmunity and Inflammation: *www.nhlbi.nih.gov/resources/chi/.*

WebMD Arthritis Health Center: *www.webmd.com/ arthritis/about-inflammation.*

Nutrition.gov (Herbal Supplements): *www.nutrition.gov/ dietary-supplements/herbal-supplements.*

University of Maryland Medical Center: *http://umm.edu/.*

American Heart Association: *www.heart.org.*

Oldways (Mediterranean diet): *http://oldwayspt.org/.*

Academy of Nutrition and Dietetics: *www.eatright.org.*

USDA Choosemyplate.gov: *www.choosemyplate.gov.*

National Sleep Foundation: *http://sleepfoundation.org/.*

SmokeFree.gov: *http://smokefree.gov/.*

National Institute of Arthritis and Musculoskeletal and Skin Diseases: *www.niams.nih.gov/Health_Info/Fibromyalgia/.*

American College of Rheumatology (Fibromyalgia): *www.rheumatology.org/Practice/Clinical/Patients/ Diseases_And_Conditions/Fibromyalgia/.*

Clean Eating: *www.cleaneatingmag.com/.*

Environmental Working Group: *www.ewg.org/.*

U.S. FDA-Good Allergies: *www.fda.gov/Food/ ResourcesForYou/Consumers/ucm079311.htm.*

U.S. Food and Drug Administration: *www.fda.gov.*

Dietary Guidelines for Americans, 2010: *www.health.gov/ dietaryguidelines.*

U.S. Department of Health and Human Service, Physical Activity Guidelines for Americans: *www.health.gov/ paguidelines/.*

Harvard Medical School, Glycemic Index and Glycemic Load for 100+ Foods: *www.health.harvard.edu/glycemic.*

Whole Grains Council: *http://wholegrainscouncil.org.*

Books

The Complete Idiot's Guide to The Mediterranean Diet (Alpha Books, 2010), by Kimberly A. Tessmer, RD, LD

Certified LEAP Therapists/Dietitians

Oxford Biomedical Technologies

http://nowleap.com/

http://nowleap.com/leap-eating-plan/ leap-anti-inflammatory-eating-plan/

Find a Certified LEAP Therapist: (866) 230-7232

Note: Many of these dietitians work via phone and can work with you from any state!

Jan Patenaude, RD, CLT

Director of Medical Nutrition

Oxford Biomedical Technologies, Inc.

Ft. Collins, CO

866-230-7232 (toll free)

Telecommuting Nationwide

Jan@CertifiedLEAPTherapist.com

http://CertifiedLEAPTherapist.com

http://PINTEREST.com/LEAPMRT

www.facebook.com/LEAP.MRT

Twitter: @LEAPMRT

Susan Linke, MBA, MS, RD, LD, CLT

Associate Director of Medical Nutrition

Oxford Biomedical Technologies, Inc.

Certified LEAP Therapist (CLT)

Dietitian/Nutritionist specializing in chronic inflammatory conditions related to food sensitivities, allergies, and intolerances.

Dallas, TX 75230

469-233-0710

www.susanlinke.com

Lea Crosetti Andes, RD, CSSD

Registered Dietitian

Board Certified Specialist in Sports Dietetics

877-66-FUEL4 (877-663-8354)

Lea@BariAthletes.com

www.BariAthletes.com

Follow BariAthletes on:

www.BariAthletes.com/blog

www.Twitter.com/BariAthleteRD

www.Facebook.com/BariAhtletes

www.Pinterest.com/BariAthletes

Dianne Rishikof, MS, RDN, LDN

617-257-3611

Natick, MA (Metrowest Boston)

dianne.rishikof@gmail.com

www.diannerishikof.com

Dana Magee RD, LD

Rebecca Bitzer MS, RD & Associates

Greenbelt & Columbia Maryland

301-474-2499

Dana@rbitzer.com

Whitney Ahneman, MS, RDN, CLT

Registered Dietitian and Certified LEAP Therapist

Serving Manhattan and Westchester County, NY

www.wittynutrition.com

www.maplemedical.com

bibliography

American Heart Association. "Inflammation and Heart Disease." Updated July 29, 2014. Accessed October 21, 2014. *www.heart.org/HEARTORG/Conditions/Inflammation-and-Heart-Disease_UCM_432150_Article.jsp.*

———. "Monounsaturated Fats." Accessed October 18, 2014. *www.heart.org/HEARTORG/GettingHealthy/NutritionCenter/HealthyEating/Monounsaturated-Fats_UCM_301460_Article.jsp.*

———. "Target Heart Rate." Updated December 2014. Accessed November 5, 2014. *www.heart.org/HEARTORG/GettingHealthy/PhysicalActivity/FitnessBasics/Target-Heart-Rates_UCM_434341_Article.jsp.*

———. "Trans Fats Q&A." Accessed December 18, 2014. *www.heart.org/HEARTORG/GettingHealthy/NutritionCenter/HealthyEating/Trans-Fats_UCM_301120_Article.jsp.*

Biesalski, H.K. "Polyphenols and Inflammation: basic interaction." *Current Opinion in Clinical Nutrition and Metabolic Care* 10, no. 6 (November 2007): 724–728. *www.ncbi.nlm.nih.gov/pubmed/18089954.*

Burris, R.L., H.P. Ng, and S. Nagarajan. "Soy protein inhibits inflammation-induced VCAM-1 and inflammatory cytokine induction by inhibiting the NF-κB and AKT signaling pathway in apolipoprotein E-deficient mice." *European Journal of Nutrition* 53, no. 1 (February 2014): 135–148. *www.ncbi.nlm.nih.gov/pubmed/23468309.*

Corti, Roberto, Andreas J. Flammer, Norman K. Hollenberg, and Thomas F. Lüscher. "Cocoa and Cardiovascular Health." *American Heart Association, Circulation* 119 (2009): 1433–1441. *http://circ.ahajournals.org/content/119/10/1433.full.*

Crofford, Leslie J. "Fibromyalgia." (Reviewed by the American College of Rheumatology Communications and Marketing Committee.) American College of Rheumatology, February 2013. *www.rheumatology.org/Practice/Clinical/Patients/Diseases_And_Conditions/Fibromyalgia/.*

Ford, E.S. "Does exercise reduce inflammation? Physical activity and C-reactive protein among U.S. adults." *Epidemiology* 13, no. 5 (September 2002): 561–568. *www.ncbi.nlm.nih.gov/pubmed/12192226.*

Franz, Mary. "Nutrition, Inflammation, and Disease." *Today's Dietitian* 16, no. 2 (February 2014): 44. *www.todaysdietitian.com/newarchives/020314p44.shtml.*

Fujii, H., M. Iwase, T. Ohkuma, S. Ogata-Kaizu, H. Ide, Y. Kikuchi, Y. Idewaki, T. Joudai, Y. Hirakawa, K. Uchida, S. Sasaki, U. Nakamura, and T. Kitazono. "Impact of dietary fiber intake on glycemic control, cardiovascular risk factors and chronic kidney disease in Japanese patients with type 2 diabetes mellitus: the Fukuoka Diabetes Registry." *Nutrition Journal* 12, no. 159 (December 11, 2013). *www.ncbi.nlm.nih.gov/pubmed/24330576.*

González, R., I. Ballester, R. López-Posadas, M.D. Suárez, A. Zarzuelo, O. Martínez-Augustin, and F. Sánchez de Medina. "Effects of flavonoids and other polyphenols on inflammation." *Critical Reviews in Food Science and Nutrition* 51, no.4 (April 2011): 331–362. *www.ncbi.nlm.nih.gov/pubmed/21432698.*

Hotamisligil, G.S. "Inflammation and Metabolic Disorders." *Nature* 444 (December 2006): 860–867. *www.ncbi.nlm.nih.gov/pubmed/17167474.*

Krishnamurthy, V.M., G. Wei, B.C. Baird, M. Murtaugh, M.B. Chonchol, K.L. Raphael, T. Greene, and S. Beddhu. "High dietary fiber intake is associated with decreased inflammation and all-cause mortality in patients with chronic kidney disease." *Kidney International* 81, no. 3 (February 2012): 300–306. *www.ncbi.nlm.nih.gov/pubmed/22012132.*

Ley, S.H., Q. Sun, W.C. Willett, A.H. Eliassen, K. Wu, A. Pan, F. Grodstein, and F.B. Hu. "Associations between red meat intake and biomarkers of inflammation and glucose metabolism in women." *American Journal of Clinical Nutrition* 99, no. 2 (February 2014): 352–360. *www.ncbi.nlm.nih.gov/pubmed/24284436.*

Libby, P. "Inflammatory mechanisms: the molecular basis of inflammation and disease." *Nutrition Reviews* 65 (December 2007): 140–146. *www.ncbi.nlm.nih.gov/pubmed/18240538.*

Lotto, V., S.W. Choi, and S. Friso. "Vitamin B6: a challenging link between nutrition and inflammation in CVD." *British Journal of Nutrition* 106, no. 2 (July 2011): 183–195. *www.ncbi.nlm.nih.gov/pubmed/21486513.*

Ma, Yunsheng, Jennifer A. Griffith, Lisa Chasan-Taber, Barbara C. Olendzki, Elizabeth Jackson, Edward J. Stanek III, Wenjun Li, Sherry L. Pagoto, Andrea R. Hafner, and Ira S. Ockene. "Association between dietary fiber and serum-C reactive protein." *The American Journal of Clinical Nutrition* 83, no. 4 (April 2006): 760–766. *http://ajcn.nutrition.org/content/83/4/760.full.*

Masters, Rachel C., Angela D. Liese, Steven M. Haffner, Lynne E. Wagenknecht, and Anthony J. Hanley. "Whole and Refined Grain Intakes Are Related to Inflammatory Protein Concentrations in Human Plasma." *Journal of Nutrition* 140, no. 3 (March 2010): 587–594. *www.ncbi.nlm.nih.gov/pubmed/20089789.*

Medical News Today. "Poor Sleep Tied to Inflammation, a Risk Factor For Heart Disease, Stroke." Last updated November 2010. Accessed October 20, 2014. *www.medicalnewstoday.com/articles/207877.php.*

Morris, Alanna, Dorothy Coverson, Lucy Fike, Yusuf Ahmed, Neli Stoyanova, W. Craig Hooper, Gary Gibbons, Donald Bliwise, Viola Vaccarino, Rebecca Din-Dzietham, and Arshed Quyyumi. "Abstract 17806: Sleep Quality and Duration are Associated with Higher Levels of Inflammatory Biomarkers: the META-Health Study." *American Heart Association, Circulation* 122 (2010): **A17806**. Accessed October 20, 2014. *http://circ.ahajournals.org/cgi/content/meeting_abstract/122/21_MeetingAbstracts/A17806.*

National Center for Complementary and Alternative Medicine (NCCAM). "Oral Probiotics: An Introduction." Last updated December 2012. Accessed October 5, 2014. *http://nccam.nih.gov/health/probiotics/introduction.htm.*

Oxford Biomedical Technologies, Inc. "How Food Sensitivities Cause Inflammation." 2013. Accessed

Nov. 1, 2014. *http://nowleap.com/food-sensitivity/ how-food-sensitivities-cause-inflammation/*.

Patenaude, Jan. "Inflammation and Food Sensitivities— Successful Treatment Begins With Patient-Centered Care." *Today's Dietitian* 13, no. 11 (November 2011): 18. *www. todaysdietitian.com/newarchives/110211p18.shtml*.

Paturel, Amy. "The Ultimate Arthritis Diet: Stock your fridge and pantry with Mediterranean staples to fight pain and inflammation." *Arthritis Foundation*. Accessed November 1, 2014. *www.arthritistoday.org/what-you-can-do/eating-well/arthritis-diet/the-arthritis-diet.php*.

Pirro, M., G. Schillaci, G. Savarese, F. Gemelli, M.R. Mannarino, D. Siepi, F. Bagaglia, and E. Mannarino. "Attenuation of inflammation with short-term dietary intervention is associated with a reduction of arterial stiffness in subjects with hypercholesterolaemia." *European Journal of Cardiovascular Prevention and Rehabilitation* 11, no. 6 (December 2004): 497–502. *www. ncbi.nlm.nih.gov/pubmed/15580061?dopt=Citation*.

Ribel-Madsen, S., E.M. Bartels, A. Stockmarr, A. Borgwardt, C. Cornett, B. Danneskiold-Samsøe, and H. Bliddal. "A synoviocyte model for osteoarthritis and rheumatoid arthritis: response to Ibuprofen, betamethasone, and ginger extract-a cross-sectional in vitro study." *J Arthritis* (2012). *www.ncbi.nlm.nih.gov/pubmed/23365744*.

Rodríguez-Hernández, H., Simental-Mendía, L.E., Rodríguez-Ramírez, G., Reyes-Romero, M.A. "Obesity and inflammation: epidemiology, risk factors, and markers of inflammation." *International Journal of Endocrinology* (April 2013). *www.ncbi.nlm.nih.gov/pubmed/23690772*.

Sandoval, M., N.N. Okuhama, X.J. Zhang, L.A. Condezo, J. Lao, F.M. Angeles, R.A. Musah, P. Bobrowski, and M.J. Miller. "Anti-inflammatory and antioxidant activities of cat's claw (Uncaria tomentosa and Uncaria guianensis) are independent of their alkaloid content." *Phytomedicine* 9, no. 4 (May 2002): 325–337. *www.ncbi.nlm.nih.gov/ pubmed/12120814.*

Simopoulos, A.P. "The importance of the ratio of omega-6/omega-3 essential fatty acids." *Biomedicine & Pharmacotherapy* 56, no. 8 (October 2002): 365–379. *www.ncbi.nlm.nih.gov/pubmed/12442909.*

van der Vaart, H., D.S. Postma, W. Timens, and N.H. ten Hacken. "Acute effects of cigarette smoke on inflammation and oxidative stress: a review." *Thorax* 59, no. 8 (August 2004): 713–721. *http://www.ncbi.nlm.nih.gov/ pubmed/15282395.*

van der Vaart, Hester, Dirkje S. Postma, Wim Timens, Machteld N. Hylkema, Brigitte W.M. Willemse, H. Marike Boezen, Judith M. Vonk, Dorothea M. de Reus, Henk F. Kauffman, and Nick H.T. ten Hacken. "Acute effects of cigarette smoking on inflammation in healthy intermittent smokers." *Respiratory Research* 6, no. 1 (March 2005): 22. *www.ncbi.nlm.nih.gov/pmc/articles/ PMC554761/.*

Wellen, Kathryn E., and Gökhan S. Hotamisligil. "Inflammation, Stress and Diabetes." *Journal of Clinical Investigation* 115, no. 5 (May 2005): 1111–1119. *www.jci. org/articles/view/25102.*

Wisse, Brent E. "The Inflammatory Syndrome: The Role of Adipose Tissue Cytokines in Metabolic Disorders Linked to Obesity." *Journal of the American Society of Nephrology* 15 (2004): 2792–2800.

Wong, Carmen P., Kathy R. Magnusson, and Emily Ho. "Increased inflammatory response in aged mice is associated with age-related zinc deficiency and zinc transporter dysregulation." *The Journal of Nutritional*

Biochemistry 24, no. 1 (January 2013): 353–359. *www.jnutbio.com/article/S0955-2863(12)00198-2/abstract.*

Zeisel, Steven H. "Is there a new component of the Mediterranean Diet that reduced Inflammation?" *The American Journal of Clinical Nutrition* 87, no. 2 (February 2008): 277–278. *http://ajcn.nutrition.org/content/87/2/277. full.*

index

about the author

Kimberly A. Tessmer, RDN, LD is a published author and consulting dietitian in Brunswick, Ohio. A few of her most recent books include *Your Nutrition Solution to Type 2 Diabetes, Your Nutrition Solution to Acid Reflux, Tell Me What to Eat If I have Inflammatory Bowel Disease, Tell Me What to Eat If I Am Trying To Conceive, The Complete Idiot's Guide to The Mediterranean Diet,* and *Tell Me What to Eat If I Have Celiac Disease.* Kim currently owns and operates Nutrition Focus (*www.nutrifocus.net*), a consulting company specializing in weight management, authoring, menu development, and other nutritional services. In addition, Kim acts as the RD on the board of directors for Lifestyles Technologies, Inc., a company that provides nutrition software solutions, developing a wide array of nutritionally sound meal templates.